CRISIS IN THE HEALTH SERVICE

CRISIS IN THE HEALTH SERVICE

THE POLITICS OF MANAGEMENT

STUART HAYWOOD
and ANDY ALASZEWSKI

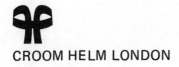

CROOM HELM LONDON

© 1980 Stuart Haywood and Andy Alaszewski
Croom Helm Ltd, 2-10 St John's Road, London SW11
ISBN 0-7099-0013-9

British Library Cataloguing in Publication Data

Haywood, Stuart, Collingwood
    Crisis in the Health Service.
    1. Health services administration-
    Great Britain
    2. Great Britain-.National Health Service
    I. Title
    II. Alaszewski, Andy
    658'.91'36210941   RA395.G6

    ISBN 0-7099-0013-9

Printed and bound in Great Britain by
Redwood Burn Limited
Trowbridge & Esher

CONTENTS

TO KAY AND HELEN

ACKNOWLEDGEMENTS

While the opinions expressed in the book remain the sole responsibility of the authors, we are pleased to acknowledge the assistance and help of many others. The empirical material is drawn from projects that have engaged the attention of a number of research staff, including Trevor James, Rick Chandler, Tad Matus, Mike Lee, Penny Clarke and Elizabeth Redmore. The encouragement of Howard Elcock and Philip Tether also merits separate acknowledgement, as does the assistance of Danny Vulliamy with preliminary versions of Chapters 2, 6 and part of Chapter 7.

Two of the three projects from which much of the material comes were the brain child of the late Ron Brown, the first Director of the Institute for Health Studies. Our debt to him is obvious, as it is to the organisations that provided the financial backing. These were the Social Science Research Council and the Nuffield Provincial Hospitals Trust. Additionally the Kings Fund College, London, also provided funds for a project initiated by Stuart Haywood and this has also influenced the content of the book. The primary debt, however, continues to be to Ron Brown whose energy led to the creation of the Institute for Health Studies and the launching of the research projects. We can only hope that the end product maintains the high standards that he set.

We are also pleased to acknowledge the ready co-operation of senior officers, members and clinicians in those health authorities which gave access to the research teams. Since we have used pseudonyms for the health authorities concerned we cannot identify the individuals whose help was especially helpful and included, in some cases, comments on drafts of particular chapters. There was nothing stinting about their responses to never-ending requests for information and opportunities for discussion.

It is customary to acknowledge the assistance of the secretary who fights her way through illegible drafts, amendments and counter amendments to produce the finished article. In this case we owe more than the usual debt to Val Hunter who achieved that magical trans-formation for us. She had the additional handicap of two authors who worked in different parts of the country at the time of the final typing. Her competence enabled her to overcome this additional obstacle with a minimum of fuss.

We should also like to thank the *Health and Social Service Journal* for permission to use much of the content of a Centre Eight Paper, 'Team Management in the NHS — What is it all about?' Finally, we acknowledge the help of our families whose younger members, in particular, showed sufficient forbearance to enable us to finish the book in reasonable time.

ABBREVIATIONS

AA	Area Administrator
AHA	Area Health Authority
AHA (T)	Area Health Authority (Teaching)
ATO	Area Team of Officers
BMA	British Medical Association
CHC	Community Health Council
DCP	District Community Physician
DGH	District General Hospital
DHSS	Department of Health and Social Security
DMT	District Management Team
GP	General Practitioner
Grey Book	Management arrangements for the reorganised NHS (1972)
HAS	Health Advisory Service
MP	Member of Parliament
NHS	National Health Service
RHA	Regional Health Authority
RHB	Regional Hospital Board
RTO	Regional Team of Officers

PREFACE

The problems of the National Health Service (NHS) continue to capture public attention. In 1979 it was the 'industrial' action of the ancillary workers unions and the relative position of NHS employees in the pay league table; in 1980 it is the effect of 'cuts' in spending and the impact of a second reorganisation of the service within a decade. Suggestions that the NHS should be financed on an insurance basis will ensure the service a continuing, prominent place in public debate in the years to come.

The affairs of the NHS merit the considerable public interest, since it is such a precious institution. Its special place in British life persists in spite of the growing attack on public welfare services and criticism is still likely to evoke responses reserved for those who attack an article of the true faith. The exception to this rule — provider complaints about the insufficiency of resources — also serves to underline the consensus about the principles of the service: the main problem is seen to be the size of the budget.

The natural pride in the NHS (which we share) and the determination to defend it from heretics, however, has had unfortunate side-effects. It tends to direct attention to external forces as explanations for difficulties. The power of the unions, the inability of the government and central department to understand the real problems of the service, the allegedly irresponsible demands of the public, and the insensitivity and number of so-called bureaucrats are among the most frequently mentioned. Closer inspection, however, suggests that these factors are scapegoats rather than causes of the more intractable problems of the NHS, such as the years of neglect of psychiatric services. The same can be said of the surprising lack of improvement in life expectancy for middle aged men, and sickness rates, escalating drug bills, the very slow development of community based services, poor manpower planning and the continued neglect of preventive medicine.

The dearth of studies of the internal dynamics of the service necessary to understand some of these developments (or the lack of them) has also undermined the effectiveness of the managerialist strategy adopted by successive governments in the last twenty years. The commitment to the idea of improvements in service by investment in management explains the considerable development of such things

11

as work study, operational research, management training, cost-benefit analysis, personnel management, restructuring of management arrangements for groups of staff and two reorganisations of health authorities. The impact of most of these developments has, or will be, less than the enthusiasts would have had us believe. One of the primary reasons for this is the assumption that the nature of NHS management, particularly the role and power of top managers, is not too dissimilar to that in private organisations from which many of the developments originate. In the absence of substantive evidence of how the management process actually worked in the NHS, the key assumptions had to be accepted at face value. Closer inspection would have revealed their inaccuracy or partiality and thus have facilitated the design of more effective change strategies.

This is why we know that the nature of the management process described in this book will survive (and perhaps even be reinforced by) the latest restructuring of the NHS.[1] The discontinuities between this set of changes and central elements in the managerialist strategy of the previous two decades are more apparent than real. Certainly there are changes of emphasis. The concerns of 1974, efficiency, defined and sophisticated managerial relations, more considered distribution of resources, are replaced by simpler, seemingly more robust notions. Simplicity is now in fashion. The management structure and planning systems are to be simplified and district health authorities are (in theory at least) to be left to do their own thing without central interference. While these will effect some changes, the essential ingredients of local management will not change: the power, values and interests of various groups will merely manifest themselves in slightly different forums.

At a more pragmatic level, the latest restructuring will not even necessarily solve some of the everyday problems to which it is expected to be particularly relevant. Many expect the simplification of the management structure, for example, to speed up decision-making. On a commonsense level, the elimination of two levels of management (area health authorities and that between district and units) should achieve this by removing some of the actors in the process. However, closer inspection suggests that the number of tiers was not the primary reason for the *additional* delays thought to have been occasioned by the 1974 management arrangements. Two more important factors were the increasing financial restraints which led to a centralisation of decision-making to effect control of spending, and the existence of a top management multi-disciplinary team. Issues with implications for other disciplines were attracted up the separate occupational hierarchies to this high level because it was multi-disciplinary: previously such issues would have been decided further down the line.[2] Similarly, the proposal to strengthen the generalist function at unit level could also have a delaying effect if functional managers now have to refer decisions, previously their own responsibility, to a general manager. Simple solutions based on popular assumptions will not alter the basic dynamics of the service.

The problems facing the NHS will, therefore, remain unaffected by the latest attempt to improve the delivery of care by rejigging the management arrangements. It is hard to see the link, for example, between the simplification of management structure and the settlement of the unrealised aspirations of professionals for more and more money, harder-headed analyses of the value of projected and current activities and the diversion of resources into those proved to have significant benefits in terms of cures and contributions to the relief of handicap. Since the strategy is based on an incomplete picture of the service, some unconsidered factor will intervene between intention and performance. Indeed the only point of significance in the latest effort for the historian in the year 2000 may well be the intensity of interest of so many highly placed people in an exercise that proved to be so peripheral to the main problems of the NHS.

If we are to do better in future, change strategies, based on a fuller appreciation of the *internal* dynamics of the NHS, have to be developed. It is no good relying on models developed in other settings or 'plain man, commonsense' assumptions. It was the disparity between such conventional assumptions and the data collected in the course of research projects conducted by the Institute for Health Studies at the University of Hull that provided the impetus for this book. We had to make sense of the empirical material. Frameworks for analysis based on conventional (and constitutionally correct) perspectives of process were found to be of little help. They did not explain much of what we found and there were few alternative studies of the NHS on which to draw. We hope the material in the book will provide a stimulus for future studies of health authorities to provide a basis for a sounder theory of the NHS.

The theme is a plea for a fresh look at the internal workings of the National Health Service to *supplement*, not replace, the insights gained in earlier studies and official commentaries. The argument is as relevant to the 'new' service (post-1980) as it is to the preceding reorganised phase, and the pre-1974 hospital management and local health committees. To underline the continuity between the old and the new, we frequently refer to health authorities as health agencies.

The purpose of the book is, however, more than understanding for its own sake. We count ourselves among the defenders of the faith as far as the NHS is concerned. The criticisms of the common assumptions about process are intended to strengthen the position of the defenders by pointing the way to more effective strategies to improve performance within the service. The more we understand about how it actually works, the easier it will be to improve the quality of service in what remains a very precious British institution.

Stuart Haywood
Andy Alaszewski

Notes

1. DHSS and Welsh Office, *Patients First* (HMSO, London, 1979).
2. S.C. Haywood, *Consensus or Constipation? A Study of Decision Making in the NHS*, a King's Fund Project Paper, Number 17 (1977).

1 THE CASE FOR A LOCAL PERSPECTIVE ON THE NATIONAL HEALTH SERVICE

The failure of the 1974 reorganisation of the National Health Service (NHS) is now widely acknowledged. The final acts of recognition came in the report of the Royal Commission in 1979[1] and the subsequent decision of the government to press ahead with further changes.[2] Although these differ from those commended by the Commissioners, the fact that they and the government were willing to change arrangements that were only five years old is a striking condemnation of the earlier reorganisation. The willingness to try again also suggests a continuing confidence in this way of promoting change in spite of the high costs of such exercises.[3]

It is not a confidence that we share. One crucial reason for the failure of the 1974 reorganisation was the false assumptions about the links between changes in structure and process, and improvements in services.[4] The latest changes share many of those assumptions and, therefore, are again likely to disappoint. On both occasions the influence and conservatism of the agencies created to deliver the services has been underestimated. Change strategies have thus been based on only partial appreciations of the dynamics of the NHS.

The theme of this book is the need for a 'local perspective' in the studies of the NHS as an essential prerequisite of a successful change strategy. The growing awareness of the weakness of governments to effect change has found some recognition in both the report of the Royal Commission and the Conservative Government's response to these proposals. While this is welcome, the previous neglect of the relationships within and between the health authorities created in 1974 means that the new strategy lacks a guidebook. Studies of health authorities are, therefore, even more urgent. They are also needed to balance the remaining 'centralist' assumptions lurking in the recantations.

The argument that a local perspective is an essential ingredient of a balanced view of a service is equally applicable to other parts of British public administration. (It is also even more germane in other Western countries in which government is playing an increasing role in the provision of health care.) In recent years studies of local authorities in Britain have underlined the importance of looking at them in their own right and not as agents of central government.[5] The assumption that the seeming legal, constitutional and financial dependence on central government meant little local room for manoeuvre has now been very effectively challenged. The interest in how local preferences arise and find expression in local authorities has not, however, been matched in the case of the NHS.

The more obvious agency status of health authorities than that of their counterparts in local government may be held to diminish the force of the argument in the case of the NHS. Health authorities are totally dependent on the central exchequer for funds while local government raises some of its own. However, it would be unwise to assume that the seemingly greater financial dependence and the stronger constitutional position of the Secretary of State *vis-à-vis* health authorities means their room for manoeuvre is limited to what the centre will concede. Evidence suggests that their preferences are very influential, that they are able to act upon them in an effective way, and central policies are not always given precedence when there is a conflict of priorities.

The case for change within the NHS is accepted without much argument in this book. We accept that changes are required in the way things are done in many authorities. Processes often manifest the dysfunctions of hierarchy and the policy of maximum consultation, without the compensating benefits. We also accept the case for a change in the balance of activities within the NHS, to take account of the growing problem of chronic rather than acute illness exacerbated by the increasing number of the very old in our population, and to redress the years of neglect in the psychiatric hospitals. The likely continuation of the present financial restrictions also requires a stronger commitment to low-cost solutions (including community care) than is the case at the moment. The problem is the development of change strategies that will facilitate these changes and reflect differences in performance. The universal prescriptions will no longer do. Do we seriously want, for example, to follow the latest change in policy – decentralisation – to its logical conclusion and decentralise to authorities where another in the depressing list of scandals in long-stay hospitals has recently erupted?

The failure of many health authorities (note not necessarily all) to respond quickly enough to changing circumstances is an important strand in our argument. The case is based on the continuing overwhelming preoccupation with acute hospital medicine in spite of the changing nature of demand and evidence that some expensive medical practices produce at best only marginal returns. The policy of developing community based services as a partial alternative has similarly only produced a muted response, in spite of their presumed cost advantages in an increasingly restrictive financial climate. While the case for the shift in emphasis can be overdone, *some* change is necessary if only to contain costs and cope, for example, with the extra demands from the increasing number of elderly for services orientated to care rather than cure. If local decision-making is to be moved more firmly in this direction, better change strategies are urgently required.

A third strand in the argument is the failure of the managerialist strategy to effect these changes. The increasing importance attached to the managerial function in health care, expressed in schemes to produce better managers, better systems, better structures, has its origins in the hospital service of the early 1960s and reached its zenith in 1974. It was based on ideas developed in profit-making firms, particularly in the manufacturing sector, and these have eventually become good currency for the management of the public sector. The post-reorganisation difficulties have not diminished the strong commitment of some to this approach. The difficulties are blamed, not on the organising concepts, but on poor design or implementation of the ideas. Banham Inc., for example, took this view in his evidence to the Royal Commission.[6] We seek to show the limitations of strategies for change based on these ideas.

This brief introduction to the direction of argument is sufficient to show that a plea for a local perspective in studies of the NHS does not mean a disinterest in wider issues. Local studies are very relevant to the wider issue of relationships between people and government in Western liberal democracies. The fuller understanding of how governments actually work will increase our appreciation of the freedoms and powers of professionals in their employ; the effect of bureaucratic systems on the people who inhabit them; the pace, type and scale of change in the nature of the service offered to the client groups; and the (alleged) centralisation of authority in government. The NHS offers a rich source of material on these and other wider governmental issues, because of its considerable size, the range of occupations employed in it and the considerable social significance attached to it.

The argument in this book is very germane to two of these issues — centralisation and the relative power of bureaucrat and professional. The second issue is, of course, a practical manifestation of the problems all libe.al democracies have in reconciling the freedom of the individual and the power of the state. The problems persist whatever the type of governmental involvement in health care. In some cases government has intervened directly and taken on responsibility for the supply of services, as in the case of the NHS. In others it has contented itself largely with providing resources (e.g. Medicare and Medicaid in the USA) from which vulnerable or deprived groups can purchase care provided by a mixture of state, voluntary or profit-making agencies. In both circumstances, increased government activity changes relationships in some way because of its fundamental nature. Government action is usually directed to changing the distribution of care away from the pattern that would have been produced by market forces if left to themselves. Action implies the use of some influence, and it is this that affects the balance between the governments' executors and service providers.

The significance of health spending for the economy also makes inevitable (or at least very probable) government action to control or influence activities of providers. This is particularly so in the UK where the government itself is responsible for the supply of services. Spending on the NHS is subject to the requirements of economic management as the frequent cuts in the capital programme and the slow-down in growth rates for revenue spending in the late 1970s testify. Similarly, pay policies of successive governments have left their impact on the service.

These developments have occasioned new relationships between the centre, health agencies and providers, whether or not state provision is of long standing as in the UK. The question of the right balance has become difficult, with health agencies feeling that the centre interferes too much and the centre perhaps feeling that it has too little control over events on the ground. The way this issue is being handled in practice makes the NHS experience very relevant to the widespread concern about overgovernment and overcentralisation. It also underlines the importance of basing prescriptions for change on realities rather than myths.

The argument is developed in three phases. The first (Chapter 2) examines the major (unofficial and official) commentaries on the NHS since its creation in 1948. The purpose is to demonstrate the outline and pervasiveness of what we call the centralist perspective. Its essence is a view of the NHS in which the major issues, though worthy of study and comment, are those that affect the service as a whole. Another characteristic is the direction of the comments. They are usually addressed to the Secretary of State or his department (hereafter both are usually referred to as the central authority or the 'centre') suggesting that they are the initiators of major change.

One set of authors, however, has been omitted, and this requires a brief explanation at this point. There is no reference to the group (mostly economists) who have argued for a (partial) withdrawal of the state from the direct provision of health services and a correspondingly larger role for the private sector. The critiques received considerable publicity in the 1960s[7] but have been excluded from our summary because of their lack of influence. We were primarily interested in commentaries that reflected official views of the NHS or were discernibly influential. It is worth noting in passing, however, that like those commentaries which are discussed they share the centralists' preoccupations with issues and prescriptions that affect the entire system.

The second phase of the argument (Chapters 3 to 6) examines the internal dynamics of the NHS. We begin (Chapter 3) by looking at the limits of central influence in the context of planning. This is necessary to establish our case that health authorities have sufficient room for manoeuvre to make studies of them worthwhile. We also explore the attempt to change the balance between services and the limitations of the managerialist approach to the problems and development of the NHS.

The scene is thus set for the examination (Chapters 4 to 6) of the various influences on the nature of health authorities. One of these influences is, of course, the formal arrangements that all authorities are required to adopt. The significance of these provisions in the post-1974 settlement is first explored by contrasting them with the likely impact of local environmental factors (Chapter 4). This is followed by an analysis (in Chapter 5) of the role of top managers, to see whether it does in fact correspond to the one specified in the blueprints. The conclusion that there is little correspondence leads us to look at the activities of medical staff (in Chapters 5 and 6) to emphasise their dominance, in what we see as a political rather than a managerial system.

An examination of *general* influences (management arrangements for the NHS, clinicians) might seem to be inconsistent with our plea for *local* studies. It is not — because the plea is directed to the point of analysis, i.e. local agencies to obtain a better understanding of their impact on the system. We also argue that the 'mixes' will differ between authorities. In other words, a particular feature may have more or less impact in different areas. The product of these mixes will be different views on appropriate process and priorities, though the general picture is likely to be dominance by acute hospital consultants.

This view of intra- and inter-authority relations brings notions of power, ideology and interest to the forefront of the analysis. This is not to say that we regard health agencies as in a perpetual state of conflict. They are not. We merely suggest that these features are essential ingredients in the local mix and analyses of health authorities have to take them into account. The implications of our material for these (and other) notions and their usefulness in helping us understand health authorities is a subject to which we return at the end of the book. In the meantime, however, some *preliminary* definitions are required to provide a framework for the passing comments on these issues in the earlier descriptions of the way the NHS actually works.

Power

'Power implies an ability to bring about some changes in the behaviour of people. In a social context it may be defined as "the capacity of an individual, or a group of individuals to modify the conduct of other individuals or groups in the manner which he desires and to prevent his own being modified in the manner in which he does not".'[8]

Our interest is those areas of activity where there is some difference of opinion between individuals or groups, based on values or interest. The way in which differences, when they arise, are handled and resolved tells us a lot about power within and between health authorities and the Department of Health and Social Security (DHSS). It is also worth remembering that power is used to obstruct change as well as promote it.

Interest

Greenwood *et al.* have recently developed helpful definitions of interest and values in the context of studies of the budgetary process,[9] though we also refer to both in non-resource contexts. They use the concept of interest in the sense of a 'motivation to defend or enhance particular organisational resources'. The resources in their paper include 'capital and revenue finances, staffing, accommodation, status and information necessary for the completion of functional responsibilities'.

Values

Values are defined as 'the commitments of a group to key sets of ideas which act as yardsticks or criteria for the appraisal of organisational operations'. The ideas (and therefore commitments) about what an authority should or should not be doing will vary between groups.

The third phase (Chapter 7) is a discussion of the significance of our argument for future studies and change strategies. The observation that the nature of decision-making in health agencies is predominantly political does not tell us what kind of political system it is. In Chapter 7 we examine this question and the light it throws on questions of power in health care organisations. Finally, we argue for a change strategy that recognises differences between health agencies (of whatever type).

Only one final introductory point now remains to be made. The field work in a series of research projects stretching from 1972 has taken us to a great number of health authorities in the North of England. The considerable variations between them were a testimony to the importance of the nature of the local system since national arrangements could not account for the differences. Yet there was little material on which to draw to explain some of the things that we found. This was the starting point for the argument here that a local perspective is a crucial element in a fuller understanding of the dynamics of the NHS.

Notes

1. Royal Commission on the National Health Service, *Report*, Cmnd. 7615 (HMSO, London, 1979).

2. DHSS and Welsh Office, *Patients First* (HMSO, London, 1979).

3. R.G.S. Brown, S. Griffin and S.C. Haywood, *New Bottles: Old Wine?* (Institute for Health Studies, University of Hull, September 1975).

4. S.C. Haywood, A. Alaszewski *et al.*, 'The Outcome of NHS Reorganisation', *Public Administration Bulletin* (Autumn 1979).

5. J. Stanyer, *Understanding Local Government* (Fontana/Collins, London, 1976).

6. J. Banham, *Realising the Promise of a National Health Service*, submission to the Royal Commission on the National Health Service, January 1977.

7. For an excellent analysis of this debate see A.J. Culyer, *Need and the National Health Service* (Martin Robertson, London, 1976), Ch. 7.

8. B. Smith, *Policy Making in British Government* (Martin Robertson, London, 1976), p. 16.

9. R. Greenwood, C.R. Hinings and S. Ranson, *The Politics of the Budgetary Process in English Local Government*, paper presented to a Political Studies Association Conference, Nottingham, March 1976.

2 PERSPECTIVES ON THE ORGANISATION AND DELIVERY OF HEALTH CARE: 1948 to 1980

This chapter is a historical background to the main analysis. In it we will show how and why a centralising managerialist perspective has come to dominate thinking about the NHS. It is our main hypothesis that this perspective has prevented an adequate analysis of local health agencies. Without this alternative, local perspective attempts to change, reform and improve the service are bound to fail.

The centralist perspective is based on a preoccupation with the activities and the agendas of central authorities – the Secretary of State for Social Services, the Department of Health and Social Security (formerly the Ministry of Health) and the national leadership of the various interest groups (staff associations, trade unions and voluntary organisations). The constitutional myth that the Secretary of State is responsible for and provides the whole service is treated as a reality. The NHS is seen as a single integrated organisation animated by the instructions of the centre. Differences in service provision, resource allocation etc. are seen as recalcitrance or mere aberrations that require improved central control.

The analyses of the NHS fall neatly into three phases. The first, which we call the formative phase, takes us up to 1960. It is dominated by the creation of an integrated hospital service and concern about rising costs. The second phase (to 1968) is dominated by ideas about management organised around the idea of a District General Hospital (DGH) and standard packages of service for a defined population. The final phase takes us into the mid-1970s and encompasses the period of reorganisation. Managerial efficiency remains an important theme but is now associated with the achievement of broader social objectives, particularly the distribution of resources between different geographical areas, social and client groups. A fourth phase of disillusionment with reorganisation has, at the time of writing, to develop a positive character, but the chapter ends with a review of current thinking about the NHS.

The Formative Period: 1948-60

The formative period is well-trodden territory, since the radical nature
of the NHS inevitably provoked widespread interest. The (then) current
perceptions of the service and its problems, are consequently well
established. The welding together of hospitals with different types of
ownership, management and traditions did not prove an easy task, the
geographical variations in the levels of service were considerable and the
initial costs were much higher than had been estimated. In the first and
second years of the service, supplementary estimates had to be
approved by the House of Commons. It was this last problem that gave
rise to the first comprehensive review when the newly elected Conservative Government set up a committee of enquiry into the cost of the
service in 1951.

The committee provided a platform for Abel-Smith and Titmus who
demonstrated that, contrary to popular opinion, the cost of the NHS
had fallen from 3¾ per cent to 3½ per cent of Gross National Product
between 1949/50 and 1953/4.[1] Their main criticism was not the rise
of NHS expenditure, but its nature. Spending was mainly on revenue
items with very little capital expenditure, although approximately 45
per cent of all hospitals were originally erected before 1891 and were
deteriorating rapidly.[2] Abel-Smith and Titmus argued for increased
spending utilising an economic model of the relationship between it
(investment) and current expenditure (consumption):

> current costs are incurred for benefits immediately obtained, while
> capital costs are for benefits which go on accruing after the end of
> the accounting period.[3]

The argument that increased capital expenditure would, in the long
term, reduce current costs was made even more explicit in an appendix
to their report entitled 'The Use of Capital Expenditure to Save Current
Expenditure'. In their view, antiquated hospital design made medical,
nursing and ancillary work inefficient and the construction of purpose-
built hospitals would lead to a considerable saving in staff and money.
The committee of enquiry, while accepting the case for increased
capital expenditure felt (correctly) that most of it would increase run-
ning costs.

The majority of the committee rejected the idea of substantial
reform, feeling that it was too early for a major reorganisation. In so
doing, they rejected changes that were to become the basis of the 1974

reorganisation, including the integration of the three branches of the NHS and teaching hospitals into the main administrative framework of the hospital service. The reasons for the last recommendation are of some interest, since they highlight the committee's assumptions about the nature of the service as a whole.

> It seems to us that one of the dangers of a national hospital service lies in over-standardisation and uniformity. There is a distinct advantage therefore in preserving the separate status of the teaching hospitals outside the Regional Hospital Board framework. In the past, the great advances in medical techniques and knowledge have come from the teaching centres, and those benefits have accrued therefore to the non-teaching hospitals.[4]

In this argument they assume, first, that the teaching hospital model of technology, curative medicine, is the correct one for the whole hospital service, and second, that the medical profession should determine the pattern of provision. The reasons for the non-consideration of alternative modes of provision included the statement, 'we know of no wide fields in which large sums of money might be expended at the present moment in order to bring preventive health services more "into line" with the curative services'.[5]

The exclusion of issues of effectiveness and other ways of organising services was balanced by an emphasis on efficiency though with a recognition of the problems involved. 'It is one of the problems of management — and a particularly difficult one in the case of the hospital service — to find right indices for measuring efficiency.'[6] Sir John Maude (in one of two minority reports) put the issue of centralisation/ decentralisation on the agenda and pointed to the peculiar hybrid organisational form of the service — ministers accountable to Parliament for services provided by agencies with varying degrees of autonomy. The consequent 'whole system' problems to which he drew attention, included the minister's role, the relationship between Regional Hospital Boards and Hospital Management Committees and the gap between those who provide the money (the Treasury) and those who spend it (the minister's agents). Maude also attacked the tripartite division of responsibility, believing that administrative structure had a clear impact on the nature of service provision.

> The mischiefs to which the division of the Service gives rise fall broadly under two heads (a) the administrative divorce of curative

from preventive medicine and of general medical practice from hospital practice and the overlaps, gaps and confusion caused thereby and (b) the predominant position of the hospital service and the consequent danger of general practice and preventive and social medicine falling into the background.[7]

Although effectiveness was 'on the agenda' in this minority report, it was in the context of administrative structure for the service as a whole, i.e. if you get that right, other things come right. This assumption was, of course, to become a key one some 20 years later in the 1974 reorganisation.

By the mid-1950s, with the traumatic birth period over, the service had settled down, much of the political fervour had been dissipated and the scene was set for non-partisan assessment of the performance of the NHS. A very influential one came from an American observer, Harry Eckstein.[8] He found much to admire in the NHS, including the unification of the hospital service, its abolition of charges at the point of delivery and a limited equalisation of resources, especially in the distribution of general practitioners. In his opinion, given the inherited problems of the NHS and initial underestimation of costs, the service was on the right course but a lot remained to be done. Eckstein suggested an injection of capital, especially in hospitals and in general practice (health centres), and reform of the tripartite structure of the service.

His main concern was efficiency rather than the effectiveness of the service. Eckstein dismissed suggestions that health care could be delivered in a different, more effective way, arguing that there had been little wrong 'with the hospitals which more of them, co-ordinated planning, and a certain amount of up-grading could not cure'.[9] His perception was of health care as a technical task, with the medical profession as its most skilled technicians. Therefore, they had the right, within the principles of equitable access, of determining not only the means but also the ends of the service.

Important ingredients in the centralist perspective are clearly apparent in this brief appraisal of Eckstein's view of the NHS. He was concerned to judge the *whole* system and makes comments on that. His prescriptions, like those of Maude, were likewise intended to be universally applicable. Abel-Smith, Titmus and the Guillebaud Committee similarly were constrained by terms of reference to debate the universal issue that captured policy-makers' attention at that time. The remedies (including leaving well alone) and the growing concern with efficiency rather than effectiveness were also directed to the central authorities for attention.

The Managerial Period: 1960-8

Although the seeds of managerialism are present in the work of Abel-Smith and Titmus, Guillebaud and Eckstein, they found purer expression in the government's Hospital Plan published in 1962. It was based on the nationally endorsed provision of a standard package of services in a standard format, the DGH. The assumption of optimal effectiveness *if* the package was efficiently operated, underlines the concern with the (universal) means rather than the ends of the NHS.

The limited capital investment between 1948 and 1962 had been largely devoted to the maintenance of the existing stock of hospitals. The Hospital Plan signalled the end of this period and the start of an era of investment for replacement and modernisation, with £500 million earmarked for capital expenditure over the next ten years. The plan was to provide the framework for this development: 'individual decisions will in future be taken not in isolation but in the context of known broad intentions for the development of the services as a whole'.[10] The key was the DGH which was to become the basic unit for the delivery of secondary care, with a standard package of services for defined catchment areas.

> In recent years there has been a trend towards greater interdependence of the various branches of medicine and also an increasing realisation of the need to bring together a wide range of facilities required for diagnosis and treatment. Hence the concept of the district general hospital . . . which provides treatment and diagnostic facilities both for in-patients and out-patients and includes a maternity unit, a short stay psychiatric unit, a geriatric unit and facilities for the isolation of infectious diseases . . . The size of the hospital this concept implies would normally be of 600-800 beds serving a population of 100,000-150,000.[11]

The authors of the plan were more optimistic than the Guillebaud Committee about the impact of capital investment on current costs. They predicted that the current expenditure would be little more since the new system would reduce expenditure through rationalisation of provisions, economies of scale and the lower maintenance costs of new buildings. Extra expenditure would come from the improved standard of care to the patients.[12] The increased cost to the patient in longer travel times were seen as a small price to pay for the additional benefits that would accrue.

The authors were aware that the expected economies could be frittered away by inefficient operation of the new system. They saw their report as the first in a whole series, with the others concentrating on the staffing and operation of the new system. The emphasis was on staff rather than patients becase it was the former that create expenditure, either directly through their pay and salaries or indirectly through their use of resources. Thus the 1962 Hospital Plan was followed by a series of reports examining the organisation of nurses,[13] ancillary workers[14] and doctors.[15] These reports culminated in the so-called Grey Book that outlined the managerial arrangements for the reorganised NHS.[16]

A close look at only the Salmon Report on senior nursing staff will suffice for our purposes since the others come from the same stock of ideas. (The reports on medical management are also discussed in detail in Chapter 7.) The assumptions in the Salmon Report also form a logically consistent world view (or, in this specific case, view of the health service) of which the central tenets were:[17]

(i) health care organisations are the same, or at least share characteristics with other large-scale, complex organisations, including industrial ones;

(ii) principles of economic rationality (including efficient utilisation of resources) are applicable to health care organisations;

(iii) there is a division between organisational members who do the work (clinicians, ward nurses etc.) and managers who provide the resources, or conditions in which the work can be done; and

(iv) implicit in this division of labour is the view of the organisation and management as the means to the clinical end. The sphere of management is organisational efficiency, and that of clinical work is effectiveness. Thus clinical ends, involving value judgements, should be made by clinicians, whereas management is seen as a value-free means to these ends.

This view contrasted strongly with the traditional view of health care organisations as unique and totally different from other types of complex organisations, especially industrial ones. Health care had been seen as lying outside the sphere of the ordinary economic relations in which private and industrial organisations were engaged. The absolute value given to the preservation of life, the presence of pain and death, the care rather than cash relationship between provider and patient, and the vocational element in employment were all seen to preclude managerial models, based on experience in organisations working to totally different terms of reference. The corollary was a view of organisation as unimportant and the uniqueness of health care institutions and the relationships with the communities they served.

The Salmon reform of the organisation of nursing staff was a move away from this view and followed logically from the nationalisation of the hospitals and the introduction of uniform conditions of service. It also represented a move away from the charismatic leadership of matrons to the bureaucratic control of nursing officers. The remit of the matrons had been very extensive with Abel-Smith according them 'absolute power' over the nurses 'reinforced by the para military organisation of the nursing staff and the rigid discipline imposed in the training schools'.[18] The matrons were also to lose this tight control of the training school in the drive for a specialist management function.

The Salmon Committee recommended separate divisions for teaching and their proposals were later developed in the Briggs Committee's deliberations on nursing.[19] Salmon also underlined the split between management and clinical work. Senior nurses who 'rolled up their sleeves' to help in the wards were told that they were often satisfying their own needs rather than offering a 'service to patients or ward sisters'.[20] Management was a specialist function in its own right, and abilities in this area, rather than a range of nursing qualifications, were commended as the qualification for the 'top' jobs.[21]

Other features of the Salmon arrangements that correspond to managerial models developed elsewhere were its hierarchal structure and the allocation of responsibilities. Three levels were created, with the top one given the job of policy-making and the middle and first-line managers responsible for its execution. The functions associated with nursing were thus divided not only vertically (nursing, teaching) but horizontally between workers and managers and within the ranks of management itself. Equally significant was the pre-eminent place given to the manager rather than the clinical nurse or trainer and the belief that the model was applicable to the *hospital* (not particular hospitals) nursing service. The managerial and centralist perspectives had thus come together.

The effect of this reform was to create a discontinuity between managers and practitioners, since the former draw on a body of knowledge outside nursing practice.

background discipline and nursing knowledge are becoming less important compared with 'abstract' managerial abilities that transcend local peculiarities and idiosyncrasies. It is increasingly the case that nursing background is required less for its utility than to legitimise the position of managers over a workforce, many of whom have frustrated professional aspirations . . . The Salmon reform over-emphasised the importance of managerial changes in job content to the detriment of clinical changes. It created a formal structure in which power, prestige and remuneration increased with distance from the point of patient contact.[22]

There have been subsequent (adverse) developments that can be associated with this change in the management of the hospital nursing service. The rift between managers and practitioners can be linked with the growth of (TUC-affiliated) union membership among nurses and has made traditional professionalism more difficult to maintain. The tradi-tional nursing professional association in the late 1960s made a limited but significant shift in the direction of trade unionism. There has also been an increased emphasis on the cash nexus, and a devaluation of the traditional vocational aspect of nursing. For example, the Salmon Report was followed by a substantial pay claim for the new grades. This was referred to the Prices and Incomes Board which endorsed the new model for nursing and gave a further push to the cash nexus.[23] It is from this period that the considerable growth in nursing militancy, with an increase in the number of so-called industrial actions, originates.

The response to the growth of industrial unrest (now not *a* problem but *the* problem of the NHS), has been remedies intended to reinforce, formalise and routinise the rift between management and workers. This is clear in the evidence of the Advisory, Conciliation and Arbitration Service to the Royal Commission on the NHS in which both sides of the management/worker divide are castigated. Neither 'a considerable proportion of managers [nor] the shop stewards with whom they deal' are considered to have the skills required in industrial relations. Improved training so that both sides can manage the divide routinely and efficiently, was recommended. For managers the 'prime' training need was said to be 'the skills of both man-management and the handling of management-union relationships, particularly at supervisor level'. On the union side, it was similarly 'the diplomatic skills of management-union relationships'.[24]

This brief discussion underlines the distance between the tradi-tional model of relationships in health care and the philosophy of the Salmon Report and the subsequent response to industrial relations problems. More germane for our purpose, however, is the light it throws on an official perspective on the NHS. The problems, solutions and developments continue to be seen in whole system terms. The growing consensus (at least among central policy-makers and leaders of professional groups) was that the primary 'problem' was (in)efficiency and widespread changes were needed to tackle it. The advocates (e.g. the leaders of the nursing profession in the case of Salmon) also continued to address their case to the central authority to get this change implemented.

The interest and preoccupation with models of organisation based on concepts developed in the private, and particularly the manufacturing, sector was not confined to providers and officials. It also informed a major academic contribution to the study of the NHS during this period. The Hospital (later Health Services) Organisation Research Unit, sponsored by the Ministry of Health and the North West Metropolitan Regional Hospital Board was established at Brunel University in 1967. The work of the unit indicates that they accepted official concern with the efficiency of the hospital organisations as their objective, though this was — as far as we know — never quite so explicitly stated. Indeed the unit operated very much on a consultancy basis, examining relationships defined as problematic by those responsible for service provision.

> All project activities, both fieldwork and training, are guided by steering committees on which are represented both members of hospital service and researchers . . . It is for the local steering committee . . . to decide which particular projects shall be undertaken and with what priority.[25]

The first major publication is similarly totally preoccupied with issues of efficiency, especially clarification of organisational roles and relationships. The delivery of health care is converted into a series of problems of co-ordination (and therefore organisational design).

> Any sizeable health organisation which employs members of a variety of occupations or professions at a number of wide-spaced sites, is likely to face certain common problems of co-ordination.
>
> > (1) It must somehow effectively co-ordinate the continuing treatment for the individual patient . . . (*co-ordination of the individual case*).
> > (2) It must effectively co-ordinate the planning and provision of services as a whole, for categories of patients . . . (*co-ordination*

of the 'patient-group').

(3) It must effectively co-ordinate the work, training, and development, of particular occupations or professional groups (*occupational co-ordination*).

(4) It must effectively co-ordinate all activities . . . at any one
particular institutional site (*institutional co-ordination*).

(5) It must effectively co-ordinate the development and provision of services as a whole, for the authority as a whole (*overall
operational co-ordination*).[26]

Since the problems of health care are defined in organisational terms,
then the solutions must also be of the same order. The Brunel Unit has
produced a healthy crop of organisational concepts (and diagrams) in
their search for better co-ordination through the clarification of roles
and relationship, of which perhaps the best known is 'monitoring'.
The development of traditional managerial hierarchies in the health
service, when the majority of relationships in the NHS are either
between autonomous practitioners or across disciplinary boundaries,
posed obvious conceptual problems. The 'solution' (based on observed
behaviour) was the concept of a monitoring role which

> arises where it is felt necessary to ensure that the activities of Y con-
> form to adequate standards in some particular respect, and where a
> managerial, supervisory or staff relation or staff relationship is
> impossible or needs supplementing.[27]

Some of the organisational concepts were fed back into the debate
on the management arrangements for the reorganised NHS. 'Scrutiny of
the Grey Book will make it clear how much the Brunel contributions to
the formulation of these management arrangements arose from the
material described in the present book.'[28]

This summary of the Brunel contribution to the period leading up to
reorganisation of the NHS, though brief is, nevertheless, sufficient to
link the unit's work with the official view of *the* problem for the NHS.
Both accepted that the need was to improve the efficiency of the
management of the service. This point, however, hardly needed making
given the unit's reputation and influence within the service. The brief
substantiation of the obvious was necessary to enable us to tie the
unit's work more closely with the centralist perspective that has dominated work and studies of the NHS since its creation.

The unit's observations were based on relationships unearthed and found helpful by *particular* health authorities involved in the consultancy and research work. In its own publications, the unit would also mention alternative arrangements that had been adopted in different settings and its staff always emphasised the advisory nature of their role. Decisions were the responsibility of the health agency or when they were involved in the discussions about the formal management arrangements for the reorganised service, the government of the day.

Nevertheless, we put the work of the unit firmly in the centralist tradition and not only because it accepted the central definition of the important issue for the NHS. It also assumes the top downwards model of organisational functioning. This is, of course, a taken-for-granted feature of private and many public organisations, as is the associated notion of overall direction from above (though no doubt presented as based on consent in this democratic age). Not only does the unit, therefore, accept the agenda of the central perspective, it also accepts the associated view on how things are (perhaps should be) done in organisations.

The Unit's descriptions of the NHS are not only partial in the sense that any study looks at only part of the whole. They are also deficient in that they assume a way of working that convincingly explains only one dimension – the contribution of the centre and its perceptions of what is important and appropriate process. It is a criticism that has also been made by others.

> Almost unbelievably, the Brunel Unit neglected to consider the effects of organisation on patients for the simple reason that 'for our purposes patients are not part of the organisation'. Concentrating on certain aspects of authority in the formal organisation, this Unit also fails to discuss the numerous interchanges which a hospital makes with its particular social environment and the interaction between various interest groups of differing power which form the very core of a hospital's social existence. The place of unions and the growing numbers of people they represent appear to have been 'almost wilfully neglected'.[29]

The second phase of the NHS from 1962 to 1968 was thus characterised by a concern with organisational, especially hospital, efficiency. This concern can be traced back to the programme of large-scale capital investment initiated by the 1962 Hospital Plan. If the investment was to pay off in reduced costs and/or improved output (patient care), then it was important that the benefits were not frittered away through inefficient management. The traditional view of health care as outside normal economic and managerial relations was accordingly replaced by a managerial perspective, based on models derived from industrial organisations. The standard package of services (the Hospital Plan) was to be supplemented with a standard package of management structures and in this development the centre was supported and guided by the Brunel Unit, in particular. The 'movement' found full expression in the 1974 reorganisation of the NHS which, however, we examine as a separate phase. The apogee of managerialism also serves to demonstrate its weaknesses as a way of understanding the dynamics of the NHS, and therefore the inadequacy of its prescriptions.

The Period of Reorganisation : 1968-74

The extension of the managerialist philosophy in the management arrangements for the reorganised NHS are sufficiently well established by now to need no repetition. Arrangements developed particularly in the pre-1974 hospital service were extended to include general practitioner and community health services. There were also formal arrangements for co-ordination with local authority Personal Social Services Departments. Some of the 'machinery' was refined to take latest thinking into account.

The 'accepted' view of how the NHS (should) works came together in the plethora of documentation produced at the time. There were two Green Papers (1968 and 1970) issued to provide a basis for discussion on the form the new service should take: they followed a decision in principle to reorganise the NHS. There was a consultative document issued by the new Conservative Secretary of State, Sir Keith Joseph, in 1971, with the White Paper outlining the forthcoming legislation in the following year. Additionally there was the Grey Book (to which we shall have many occasions to refer), outlining the management arrangements for the new service (1972), and much later (1976) the guide to the new planning system. The quantity of available material provides us with an authoritative and comprehensive official view of the NHS and thus ample information to substantiate our argument of the pervasiveness of an inadequate centralist/managerialist (the two reinforce each other) perspective on its dynamics.

There was, however, a second element that had been absent in the managerialism of the 1960s. A concern about the *outputs* of the service signalled a growing interest in effectiveness as well as efficiency.

In the Hospital Plan and the associated managerial reforms the emphasis was on more rational decision-making for its own intrinsic value (and possibly for cost control). The scandals in the chronic and mental sectors during the 1960s facilitated a firm set of objectives for the reorganised system – a better balance between the alternative forms of care, and redistribution of resources in terms of geographical areas and client groups.[30] Thus the means – a more rational and efficient managerial structure and decision-making system – were given firmer ends to which to work.

The rediscovery of the issue of effectiveness changed the focus of the centralist view of the NHS. It did not, however, change the view of how the service does or should operate. The concern was with the effectiveness of the service *as a whole* – as indicated by how it attacked the relative deprivation of particular sectors – and the response was another *general* prescription. While there was a growing realisation of the weakness of the centre to influence events in the NHS, the top downwards model of direction (based of course on consent) continued to guide official responses and informed comments in discussions of effectiveness.

Reorganisation and Effectiveness of Health Services

The second Green Paper on reorganisation, published in 1970, contained a clear statement on a policy objective for the NHS. It was the promotion of a more equitable distribution of resources by a shift from the better-off services and areas to the neglected and under-financed ones. This was necessary to realise a fundamental principle of the NHS:

> the same high quality of service . . . should be provided in every part of the country . . . Further levelling up of resources . . . is needed to provide the same high quality of service all over England. There are also unjustifiable differences between the average standards of care provided for long-stay hospital patients – the elderly, the mentally ill and the handicapped – and the standards of care of the short-stay hospital patients. In the services paid for partly from local rates, standards of services also differ.[31]

Sir Keith Joseph, the next Secretary of State, although of a different political persuasion, made much the same point in his foreword to the 1972 reorganisation White Paper.

There were also discontinuities between Crossman (in office in

1970) and Joseph that are germane to our argument. Crossman was
more interested in the NHS as a tool of social reform. For example, he
was especially concerned about the apparent inability of ministers to
shift resources away from the medical 'glamour' areas, the high technology acute hospitals orientated primarily to cure rather than care objectives, to the neglected areas such as the long-stay institutions and
primary care. Joseph's proposals were more concerned with managerial
efficiency, the means rather than the ends. Although he endorsed Crossman's priorities, his distinctive contribution, according to his own
claim, was the emphasis on effective management in which scientific
management structures and processes were to be a significant element.
Nevertheless, the priorities remained as the objective to which the
service would work and the formal management arrangements were part
of that grand design. The notion of a grand design for universal application is, of course, another product of thinking of the NHS as a unitary
system, which in turn has been linked with the centralist perspective
on how it works.

The reorganisation documents raise many other issues. We are concerned however only to tease out the expected relationships between
formal elements in the new arrangements and desired behaviours. This is
necessary as a basis for comparison in our later analysis of how health
authorities actually work. It also reinforces our argument that the
'wholeness' of the reorganisation package is another illustration of the
centralist perspective at work. This in turn enables us to underline
features of this perspective as a prelude to pointing to their weaknesses
both as explanations of events and thus a basis for prescription.

Not all the changes are equally cogent to the concepts of efficiency
and effectiveness that provide the rationale of reorganisation. There were
other considerations, not the least of which was the acceptability of
proposals to the groups affected by them. Clearly, the strength of the
link between *each* element in the formal arrangements and the objectives of change would have been expected to vary. At the very least,
however, we can surmise that the elements were not intended to be
inimical to those objectives: they would have to pass the test of
minimal compatibility with them. We therefore confine our discussion
to changes that were most central to the grand design of reorganisation.

Administrative Unification. The case for ending the tripartite division
of responsibility for health services was said, from the outset, to be
something more than a wish for administrative tidiness. The division
was seen as a major obstacle to a change in the balance of priorities. The

first Green Paper (1968) had said that the tripartite structure limited 'the range of those responsible for planning future progress to their own segment of the service'.[32] It went on to say that these divisions must not be allowed to reappear in the new health boards. The second Green Paper (1970) argued that the division of responsibility between dfferent agencies made it 'difficult' for them to take fully into account 'the advantages . . . to the health service as a whole' when decisions had to be made on the 'priority to give to their health services against the competing needs of their other services'.[33] The creation of one authority with responsibility for all health services was expected to remove this barrier, promote comprehensive analysis and widen choices.

Change in the Relationship between the Centre and the Periphery. In spite of his criticism of the first Green Paper on the grounds that it would have led to a very centralised service,[34] one of Crossman's own stated aims was 'effective central control over the money spent on the service . . . to ensure that the maximum value is obtained from it'.[35] More central control was also seen to be necessary for the redistribution of health service resources and a subsequent minister put the case in the following way:

> The DHSS has . . . never appeared to give priority to the task of redressing inequalities . . . seemed instead to act as the arbiter between pulling and vociferous claims of regional hospital boards, the boards of governors of teaching hospitals and postgraduate hospitals, and the local hospital management committee . . . Such 'Cinderella areas' as mental handicap and long-stay hospital patients have been seriously neglected. Parliament and Ministers have not concentrated enough on the systematic and objective allocation of resources based on defined need in an attempt to redress inequalities of health care.[36]

Scientific Management. We have already made frequent reference to this strand in thinking and policy and we return to it (in the context of particular health authorities) in Chapter 5. At this point the reference is therefore included only for the sake of completeness. The introduction or extension of structures based on experience elsewhere can be justified as a 'good thing' in itself regardless of 'new' objectives. In this case the link between structures and objectives was the emphasis on clear lines of accountability from the grass roots of the service to the Secretary of State. This was the mechanism (an integral part of the structure) through which central priorities could be most easily realised.

Professional Participation in Management. Another strong theme in NHS reorganisation was increased professional participation in management. 'The doctor and other professional workers . . . have the opportunity . . . of playing a much greater part than hitherto in the management decisions that are taken in each area.'[37]

One interpretation of this provision is that it is potentially inconsistent with the managerial thrust of the grand design. It is suggestive of a model of decision-making involving interaction and bargaining between groups rather than the rational decision-making one implied by the other elements in the arrangements for the new service. The link comes, however, in involvement of clinicians in management and the assumption that their contribution will be shaped by that experience and thus strengthen the management function.

Structure and Process. The new arrangements were expected to change process and behaviour. The unification of hospital and community services, for example, was expected to lead fairly automatically to an integrated decision-making process, in which the needs of both were balanced against each other and the best distribution of resources examined. It was thought necessary, however, to supplement changes in structure by the introduction of new formal processes for decision-making. The most significant of these was the new planning system, foreshadowed in the White Paper (1972), to replace the one initiated by the 1962 Hospital Plan.

The impact of the new planning system is a subject to which we return in the next chapter, so we confine our attention here to those features that link it to the 'grand design' of reorganisation. It was designed to improve the quality of managerial decision-making by requiring health authority personnel to follow particular analytical processes in the preparation of plans. The processes were intended to enable planners to exploit the advantages of integration by, for example, encouraging them to consider carefully the alternatives opened up by the responsibility for all local health care facilities. The model for the sequence of thought advocated in the planning guide falls squarely in the well-known definition of rational decision-making, that starts with identification of objectives (needs) and ends with implementation and review.

The allocation of responsibilities also naturally fitted the grand design. The final decisions, after the due process of consultation and the

solicitation of advice was clearly that of senior management and the
health authority. They were the ones to set the local objectives which
would provide the framework for the activities of middle and first
line management. In short, the new planning system was the physiology
and the formal structure the anatomy of the brave new managerial
world for the NHS.

The Grand Design: 1974-6

The success of the grand design depended on the validity of the
assumptions on the nature of management in the NHS and the feasib-
ility of the kind of system it was trying to promote. The shakiness of
those assumptions are, of course, one of the themes in the remainder of
this book but one key point merits a mention here. The planning
system remains primarily concerned with inputs rather than quality of
services (outputs) and their impact on health (outcomes). There are
many reasons for this, including the difficulty of measuring the quality
of service but the implicit assumptions about the link between
standardised inputs and desired outcomes (i.e. effectiveness) are shaky
ones. The utilisation of standard 'packages' will vary from area to area
because of differences in local performance. Even a national planning
system does not in any way diminish (perhaps it even enhances it) the
significance of local managers and providers in translating resources
into effective services.

Other Contributors. The increasing interest in effectiveness was echoed
by the growing number of academic contributions in this vein during
the reorganisation period. One of the major medical contributions was
from Cochrane who expressed concern at the bland assumptions about
the benefits of some existing interventions and advocated randomised
clinical trials as a general evaluatory procedure.[38] McKeown was also
concerned to attack the assumption that all improvements in life-
expectancy have come from high-technology curative medicine. He
does not argue that high-technology medicine is useless, but rather that
its impact is limited and more attention needs to be devoted to prevention and alleviation.[39]

The non-medical critics usually have a broader perspective, being
concerned with the overall impact of the NHS.[40] One theme favoured
by the 'radicals' is that the wrong structures were being introduced in
1974 and these would have a negative effect on effectiveness.
Draper and Smart, for example, have argued that the essence of
reorganisation was increased central control over peripheral health

agencies with the introduction of industrial models of organisation as a
key element in this strategy.

> the government has concluded that control should be centralised
> and that decision makers should be appointed and answerable to
> their superiors higher up in the structure rather than to the staff . . .
> or directly to the public.[41]

This centralisation would, however, do little to alter the fundamental
balance of power since the medical profession, especially the acute
specialisms, are just as powerful centrally as they are locally. The same
realities of power would, therefore, continue to apply to the redistribution of resources geographically and between services.

They developed the argument further by asserting that reorganisation actually reinforced medical hegemony and the existing definition
of the medical task. The commitment to the high-technology hospital-
oriented curative approach to medicine was strengthened, thus
reducing the influence of alternative approaches to the medical task.
The planning system, based on a narrow, technical definition of disease
and health was one feature of the new arrangements that had this
effect. This definition was held to disregard the social and pluralistic
nature of health goals[42] and create the illusion that the expert (doctor
and/or manager) can rely on independently established or objective facts
to make rational decisions.

Another feature of the reorganised structure that systematically
reinforces the technocratic approach to health care was the role given to
public health specialists. They are seen as a (potentially) dissident group
within the medical profession, capable of balancing the dominant
individualistic/physical model of disease with a more collective/social
one. To be effective these specialists must be independent and must be
prepared to act politically. However, in the new arrangements specialists
in public health were co-opted into the main managerial structure as
DCPs (District Community Physicians) and Area Specialists in
Community Medicine. Their managerial role is made explicit in the
Grey Book. 'The specialist in community medicine must be more than
an adviser. As agreed in the Hunter Report, he must be part of the
management structure.'[43]

Towell has suggested that the managerial function of the DCP was
central to the success of reorganisation in terms of better use of clinical
resources. He was the main agent of management control, being
responsible for the co-ordination and provision of information to

clinicians, the evaluation of effectiveness of services and preventive medical personnel.[44] Draper and Smart, on the other hand, see the DCP made into a technobureaucrat and the end of his effective role of the public health specialist.

> The community physician is expected . . . to become accountable within the national management hierarchy or technobureaucracy. The unpopular voice that would sometimes speak out about questions of health and the public interest and, if need be, offend and irritate established interest groups, instead of being streng- thened, will be effectively silenced by absorption.[45]

This group of critics (not Cochrane and McKeown) are not against change strategies based on reform of structure. Draper and Smart's criticisms, for example, postulate that cetain types of organisational structures are related to certain types of outcome. The drift of their argument is not that there was an overemphasis on changes in structure and a misplaced confidence in the impact these would have on outcomes (essentially our position). It is that the *wrong* structure was selected. They advocate a decentralised structure with managers and medical practitioners accountable to local service users. 'Instead of an effective devolution of power, an adaptive decision structure, and a less hierarchical administrative plan, we are confronted with the exact opposite.'[46]

Even though Draper and Smart call for more decentralisation, their framework for analysis (and therefore their prescription) is clearly centralist. They talk about NHS as a unitary system (the doctors, the managers etc.) and advocate universal prescriptions (decentralisation). The argument is addressed to the central authorities, presumably because they are seen to be the initiators of important changes of this type. The advocacy of alternative strategies to those adopted by govern- ment is not evidence of a balanced perspective on the way the NHS actually operates.

Conclusion and Postscript

The most influential analyses of the NHS have, quite naturally, tended to view the service as a whole. Judgements have been made of the performance of the whole system and prescriptions for change have been similarly oriented. The tenor of the commentaries have reflected central concerns (cost control in the 1950s, efficiency in the 1960s, equitable distribution of resources in the 1970s) and the pleas for change have been addressed to the DHSS and Secretary of State. The growing emphasis on managerialism is an integral part of this syndrome. The centre sees the prime problem as the technical one of increasing efficiency, and scientific management structures and processes derived from the same stock of ideas are the result.

There is nothing wrong with this approach. Our argument is that it is based on a view of how the NHS works that has yet to be proved. It is far from clear, for example, that the centre has sufficient power to effect the changes the critics and improvers would like to see. It is far from obvious that what is good for Bournemouth is also good for Glasgow or that the universal remedy will have the same effect in both places. The local dimensions to NHS activity have been ignored, with the result that the analyses and prescriptions have been relevant to only one element in the mix. It is our contention that this local dimension has been seriously underestimated and it is high time that focus of attention in NHS studies changed to take it into account. Without such studies the nature of the activity *within* (not of) the NHS will be so imperfectly understood that the gross errors in the reorganisation of 1974 could be repeated.

There is evidence of a rethink at the time of writing but the early signs are not too encouraging. This fourth phase of thinking about the NHS is developing out of dissatisfaction with the failure of the managerialist prescriptions to deliver the goods. In particular, they have failed to contain costs, prevent considerable industrial unrest, change the direction and orientation of the health care activities and the tension between the centre and the peripheral agencies has persisted. In other words, reorganisation has neither made the service more efficient (the managerialist objective) nor more effective. Furthermore, there is also a loss of confidence in further large-scale structural reforms. They are expensive. Expected savings are never achieved and the estimated costs always exceeded.

The reaction was evident in the first major policy statement of the Conservative Secretary, Mr Patrick Jenkin, in 1979:

The main thrust of our policy must be to make our NHS far more of a local service . . . my Department has come to concern itself much too much with detail. Of course, we must seek to achieve national standards of care; and of course, proper accountability must be safeguarded. But I also believe that doctors and other professional people in the NHS are trained to take professional decisions off their own bat and do not need the torrent of advice to which in recent years they seem to have been subjected. Equally, I believe that it is wrong to treat the National Health Service as though it were, or could be, a single, giant, integrated system. Rather must we try to see it as a whole series of local health services serving local communities and managed by local people, and I accept that different arrangements will be found appropriate in different parts of the country . . . Some of the recent industrial problems could I think have been avoided or mitigated if local managers had had more flexibility to manage. One of the problems of the NHS is that there is too much administration and not enough management.[47]

The sentiments are shared by the Royal Commission who have advocated an incremental change strategy with acceptance of (regional) differences. The commission also pointed to the weakness of the centre and the gap between its power to get things done and its constitutional reponsibilities. 'It is clear that there is a gap between the formal, detailed accountability that his chief officials carry for all that goes on in the NHS and every penny spent on it, and the realities of the situation.'[48] Like the Secretary of State, they nevertheless advocate some structural reform and at the time of writing multi-district Area Health Authorities (AHAs) are destined for the dustbin.

The change of emphasis, though welcome, still contains overtones of the centralist perspective. A policy of 'decentralisation' implies a positive act to give health agencies freedoms that they do not already possess. It also implies that the centre could re-acquire that power. The assumptions about the directorate role of the centre, its power and the need for universal policies (do we really want to decentralise power to hospitals where new scandals are imminent?) are all too evident in a decision to decentralise.

However, this may be thought to be looking a gift horse in the mouth. After all, the proposed changes recognise ability of health authorities to have a decisive influence on events in the NHS. The policy of decentralisation, though presented as a magnanimous act informed by a new radical philosophy of getting government off the people's backs, can also be said to recognise existing realities. The form of presentation should not, in other words, be allowed to obscure the significance of the changes. If this is so, then our case for looking at the way health authorities work is even *stronger* since their contribution to the development of health services within their bailiwick now has the seal of official recognition. The remainder of this book is intended to be a first step on this long road to a fuller understanding of what makes the NHS tick.

Notes

1. *Report of the Committee of Enquiry into the Cost of the National Health Service* (Guillebaud Report), Cmnd. 9663 (HMSO, London, 1956), paras. 20-1.

2. Ibid., para. 2(20).

3. B. Abel-Smith and R. M. Titmus, *The Cost of the National Health Service in England and Wales* (Cambridge University Press, Cambridge, 1956), p. 13.

4. Guillebaud Report, para. 731(1).

5. Ibid., para. 621.

6. Ibid., para. 731(17).

7. Ibid., p. 279.

8. H. Eckstein, *The English Health Service, Its Origins, Structure and Achievement* (Harvard University Press, Cambridge, Mass., 1964).

9. Ibid., p. 47.

10. Ministry of Health, *A Hospital Plan for England and Wales*, Cmnd. 1604 (HMSO, London, 1962), para. 49.

11. Ibid., para. 20.

12. Ibid., para. 47.

13. Ministry of Health, *Report of the Committee on Senior Nursing Staff Structure*, Chairman, B. Salmon (HMSO, London, 1966); National Board for Prices and Incomes, *Pay of Nurses and Midwives in the National Health Service*, Report No. 60, Cmnd. 3585 (HMSO, London, 1968).

14. National Board for Prices and Incomes, *The Pay and Conditions of Services of Ancillary Workers in the National Health Service*, Report No. 166, Cmnd. 4644, (HMSO, London, 1971).

15. Ministry of Health, *First Report of the Joint Working Party on the Organisation of Medical Work in Hospitals*, Chairman, Sir G. Godber (HMSO, London, 1967); Second Report 1970; Third Report 1974.

16. DHSS, *Management Arrangements for the Reorganised National Health Service* (HMSO, London, 1972).

17. In this analysis we draw on the work of Carpenter and Manson. M. Carpenter, 'The New Managerialism and Professionalism in Nursing', and T. Manson, 'Management, the Professions and the Unions' in M. Stacey *et al.*, *Health and the Division of Labour* (Croom Helm, London, 1977).

18. B. Abel-Smith, *A History of the Nursing Profession* (Heinemann, London, 1960), pp. 28-9.

19. *Report of the Committee on Nursing*, Chairman, Professor A. Briggs, Cmnd. 5155 (HMSO, London, 1972).

20. *Committee on Senior Nursing Staff Structure*, para. 1.13.

21. Ibid., para. 1.15.

22. Carpenter, 'The New Managerialism', pp. 183 and 185.

23. National Board for Prices and Incomes, *Pay of Nurses*.

24. Advisory, Conciliation and Arbitration Service, *Royal Commission on the National Health Service: ACAS Evidence*, Report No. 12 (1978), paras. 5.1 to 5.2.

25. R. Rowbottom, *Hospital Organisation. A Progress Report on the Brunel*

Health Services Organisation Project (Heinemann, London, 1973), p. 3.

26. Ibid., p. 223.

27. Ibid., p. 267.

28. Ibid., p. vi.

29. P. Draper and T. Smart, 'Social Science and Health Policy in the United Kingdom', *International Journal of Health Services*, vol. 4, no. 3 (1974), pp. 453-70.

30. *Report of the Committee on Enquiry into allegations of ill-treatment of patients and other irregularities at the Ely Hospital, Cardiff*, Cmnd. 4861 (HMSO, London, 1972). For the relationship between the Ely Report and changes in DHSS policy, especially the shift of priorities and resources from the acute to the chronic sectors, see R. Crossman, *The Diaries of a Cabinet Minister, Vol. 3* (Hamish Hamilton & Jonathan Cape, London, 1977).

31. DHSS, *The Future Structure of the National Health Service* (HMSO, London, 1970), p. 1.

32. Ministry of Health, *The Administrative Structure of Medical and Related Services in England and Wales* (HMSO, London, 1968), p. 10.

33. DHSS, *The Future Structure*, para. 12.

34. Crossman, *Diaries, Vol. 3*, p. 456.

35. DHSS, *The Future Structure*, para. 6.

36. D. Owen, *In Sickness and Health:The Politics of Medicine* (Quartet Books, London, 1976), pp. 5-7.

37. *National Health Service Reorganisation: England*, p. vii.

38. A.L. Cochrane, *Effectiveness and Efficiency* (Nuffield Provincial Hospital Trust, London, 1971).

39. T. McKeown, *The Role of Medicine* (Nuffield Provincial Hospital Trust, London, 1976).

40. The main texts we use will be Draper and Smart, 'Social Science and Health Policy'; P. Draper, G. Grenholm and G. Best, 'The Organisation of Health Care: A Critical View of the 1974 Reorganisation of the National Health Service' in D. Tuckett, *An Introduction to Medical Sociology* (Tavistock, London, 1976); and V. Navarro, *Medicine under Capitalism* (Croom Helm, London, 1976).

41. Draper and Smart, 'Social Science and Health Policy', p. 455.

42. Ibid., p. 457.

43. *Management Arrangements*, para. 4.19.

44. D. Towell, 'Making Reorganisation Work. Challenges and Dilemmas in the Development of Community Medicine' in K. Barnard and K. Lee (eds.), *Conflicts in the National Health Service* (Croom Helm, London, 1977).

45. Draper and Smart, 'Social Science and Health Policy', p. 457.

46. Draper, Grenholm and Best, 'A Critical View', pp. 278-9.

47. DHSS, 'Local Management, not Centralised Bureaucracy', Press Release, no. 79/133.

48. Royal Commission on the National Health Service, *Report*, Cmnd. 7615 (HMSO, London, 1979), para. 19.6.

3 THE POWER OF THE CENTRE IN THE NHS: THE REALITY

Introduction

The analyses of the NHS described in the previous chapter share one basic assumption: that significant power to effect change resides in the Secretary of State and the DHSS. Otherwise promises to 'decentralise' decision-making and 'devolve' authority would be seen to be emptier of substance than most policy pronouncements, and pleas for action would be addressed elsewhere. Activities of pressure groups and MPs continue to be directed at the centre rather than health authorities, though publicity could be another consideration.

The centralists have perhaps not made a sufficient distinction between responsibility (which does reside in the centre) and effective authority, though this is not true of commentators like Rudolph Klein: 'for the State to involve itself in the control of the health service is also to make itself dependent on the cooperation of those who actually deliver the service. The power of control is largely illusion . . . '[1] The notion of the authority of local personnel derived from the centre, while constitutionally correct, does not tell us much about how the NHS actually works. The centre is but one party to the process and its relative weakness has been masked by the constitutional arrangements. In this chapter we substantiate this view by exploring the *limits* of the centre's ability to influence local decisions.

The argument is developed in the context of central policies giving a higher priority than hitherto to services for the mentally ill and elderly, and a lower one for general, acute hospital and maternity services. Some might hold that this is an unfair test of central power. These policies aim to change the balance of priorities, which is a difficult operation in any organisation and, in any event, can only be judged over a long timescale. The policies — as far as the implications for acute and maternity services are concerned — only crystallised in 1976 and a three-year period could be held to be insufficient to make substantive judgements.

While there is some merit in these arguments, the implication that the centre has more power in more mundane activities is suspect. The DHSS has had difficulty in effecting change in relatively minor matters.

45

It had problems, for example, in the mid-1970s in getting health authorities to supply information about the basis on which charges for staff meals were based and getting them to charge a realistic rate. This was in spite of the interest of the Public Accounts Committee of the House of Commons.[2] Earlier, Rosemary Stewart's account of how hospital management committees responded to a departmental circular asking for examination and improvement of the management of out-patient departments demonstrated the local capacity for non-action. The title of her report, 'Continuously Under Review', illustrated a frequent tactic by which central scrutiny could be avoided while nothing was being done.[3] There is thus no real reason to think that the choice of policies on developments will give an exaggerated view of central weakness.

The objection of a too small timescale does not apply to the policies designed to give the 'cinderellas' of the NHS a higher priority. Most were of long standing, and in the case of services for the mentally ill are now approaching venerability. Also, since it is only in the late 1970s, when the actual and projected growth rates for the NHS were cut, that the implications of these preferences for other services became clear, the initial responses to this new situation are an indication of the likely impact of central policies on local decisions. The use of this policy initiative is therefore a fair test with which to tease out the limits of central power in the NHS.

The Balance Between the Centre and Health Authorities: The Impact of Reorganisation

The weakness of the centre in the first 25 years of the service was acknowledged in the 1974 reorganisation of the NHS. There were a number of features in the new arrangements that were designed to remedy the situation. The significant reduction in the number of 'local' health authorities foreshadowed in the first Green Paper (1968) was seen by Richard Crossman as a method of increasing central control over the service.[4] However, one of the main aims of his own proposals (outlined in the second Green Paper) was 'effective central control over the money spent on the service . . . to ensure that the maximum value is obtained from it'.[5] Nor did his own successor, Sir Keith Joseph, though of a different political persuasion, demur from this line of argument. He put considerable emphasis on clearer lines of accountability than hitherto from health authority personnel right through to the Secretary of State himself.

Clearer lines of accountability were not, however, the only new feature of the post-reorganisation arrangements designed to facilitate greater central control over local management activity (clinical autonomy remained unaffected). The key element was the new planning system, foreshadowed in the pre-reorganisation documents but not introduced until 1976. Under this system health authorities prepare operational (for the next three years) and strategic (for the next ten) plans, in the context of central policies. While norms of provisions (e.g. hospital bed: population ratios) and guidelines have long existed, a new feature is the promulgation of national priorities.

Previously, the centre had indicated issues and services to which they wanted health authorities to pay particular attention. The impact of these requests, in aggregate, while commending themselves to lobbyists, inevitably exceeded available resources. Under this arrangement the centre could also avoid the embarrassment of indicating which services and client groups deserved *less* priority. The Consultative Document on priorities, published in 1976,[6] therefore represented an assumption of responsibility by the centre. While it was issued for consultative purposes, its contents, including the relative priority that should be accorded to different services, were expected to inform plans currently being prepared. It was, therefore, an act of centralisation reinforced by the requirement that plans required the approval of higher authority (Regional Health Authorities (RHAs) in the case of AHAs, DHSS in the case of RHAs). The process, however, was to focus on proposals inconsistent with agreed policies. 'In short, the reviewing Authority will be responsible for ensuring, not that the plan is "right", but rather that it is not clearly wrong or inadequate.'[7]

Other features of the planning system and the new management arrangements were also designed to increase the power of the centre. It will therefore clearly not be enough to draw on pre-1974 experience to demonstrate the limits of the centre's ability to influence events in the localities. We do, however, include such examples to show that the texture of central-local relations is relatively impervious to this kind of (re)organisational engineering and that current conventional wisdoms about increased centralisation owe more to the theory rather than the practice of the new management arrangements.

Central Policies on Priorities in the NHS

DHSS policy, outlined in the 1976 Consultative Document, made it clear that a higher priority than hitherto should be accorded in local plans to, *inter alia*, services for the mentally ill and elderly, and more generally to community rather than institutional care. Since the growth rate for the NHS was lower than had been the case in the previous few years it was recognised that this could only be achieved if increases in spending on the general, acute and maternity hospital services (accounting for more than 40 per cent of the total) could be restrained. The document mentioned a growth rate of only 0.9 per cent per annum in the years to 1980 for the latter group of services compared with a figure four times higher for the period 1970/1 to 1973/4. The growth rates for services for the elderly (and physically handicapped) and mentally ill were 3.2 per cent and 1.8 per cent per annum. Both were also lower growth rates than for the immediately preceding period.

The examination of the success of the centre's policy on priorities must be based on quantitative *and* qualitative data. The latter compensates for the differential relevance of national figures (as it was realised), given the different base lines from which AHAs started, and it also provides an early warning of likely response since changes often take a considerable time to manifest themselves in quantitive data. We concentrate on the fortunes of the services for the mentally ill and elderly (beneficiaries of the 'new' policy) and maternity services (the 'losers'). The focus of attention is evidence of an alteration in their relative positions rather than the achievement of changes *within* the service itself.

Services for the Mentally Ill

Health services for the mentally ill have long been dominated by the mental hospital. However, a rethink of their role eventually led to the 1959 Mental Health Act, which reflected a desire to reduce the emphasis on detention and custody and focus attention much more than hitherto on active treatment. The advances in chemotherapy in particular had made a wider range of treatments available and the growing knowledge of the harmful effects of institutional life provided another incentive for shorter periods of treatment. The increasing interest and hope for the mentally ill was also reflected in ministerial promises that services for them would in future be given a higher priority within the NHS. These promises were made by a succession of ministers and pressed with increased vigour by Richard Crossman (1969-70) who used scandals in long-stay hospitals to effect changes.

The interest of ministers produced some positive results. In the 1960s, for example, additional money was earmarked for improving catering services (the amount spent on food had been much lower than that for the patients in acute hospitals). Another change was the creation of the Hospital Advisory Service (HAS) in 1969, whose early work was confined to services for the mentally ill, mentally handicapped and the elderly. The *relative* position of the mentally ill patient *vis-à-vis* his acute medical counterpart, however, had not improved significantly. The difference between the amount spent per week on patients in chronic and acute hospitals in 1968 was about the same as it had been 20 years earlier.[8]

The lack of relative improvement was at least partially explained by the resistance of hospital authorities. The tone of Richard Crossman's comment on the Regional Hospital Board (RHB) Chairman's reservations about a switch of 1¼ per cent of resources 'from the rest of the service to the sub-normal' makes it clear that he felt his sense of priorities was not shared.[9] While his impatience may have reflected a lack of realism about what could be achieved in the short term, it was a period of substantial growth in available resources. In these circumstances, the reservations are likely to have been more than the practical ones of timescale etc. and have been directed to the relative priorities of acute and psychiatric hospitals.

These events preceded reorganisation. However, the fate of monies earmarked for the provision of secure units for violent and particularly difficult patients does not suggest any radical change. In 1976 health authorities were given a special allocation to provide these units. Since this would take some time, and authorities had first to submit schemes for departmental approval, 'interim' units could be established. In 1979 — some three years after the process had been commenced — four RHAs had not even reached the stage of submitting outline plans, and no regional secure unit had been opened: interim units had been provided in only three regions. The monies allocated for this purpose — some £5 million plus by 1979 — had largely been absorbed into other expenditure.[10] One reason given to us for this slow or non-response by RHAs were the misgivings of trade unionists and other providers. While these were being overcome, the monies have been diverted, at least in one region, to services for the elderly and mentally ill. However, this explanation of the difficulties faced by RHAs strengthens rather than weakens our contention about central weakness in effecting change. Local views have, if this be the case, proved to be a more cogent consideration for RHAs than central wishes backed by specific monies and by MPs. In the planning guidelines for 1979/80 the DHSS had to content itself with a reminder to health authorities that the 'provision of regional secure units must continue to be given high priority'.[11]

The annual DHSS circulars reviewing progress on the implementation of plans do not make for easy comparisons from year to year. There were changes, for example, in the way expenditures were classified in the 1977 Planning Document, *The Way Forward.* [12] It is not, therefore, easy to say whether the proportion of the NHS budget allocated to services for the mentally ill has increased — as it should have done if the growth rates suggested in the 1976 Consultative Document had been followed by health authorities. The circulars do, however, contain references to changes. In 1978 we were told that 'statistics available nationally since the publication of the previous guidelines indicate that . . . staffing and other standards in psychiatric hospitals continue to rise . . . '. Nevertheless, the 'projected' growth figure for services for the mentally ill was *lower* than in the 1976 Consultative Document (for a slightly different period), while the increase for general, acute and maternity services was *higher.* [13]

On the same day, a press release rebutted allegations by the Director of the National Association for Mental Health (MIND) that the Secretary of State had been 'forced to more or less abandon previously stated priorities'. MIND had taken the view that *The Way Forward* had represented a watering down of the priorities accorded to services like those for the mentally ill in the previous year's Consultative Document. While the exchange centred on proposals rather than performance, it demonstrates the doubts that groups like MIND harbour about priorities in practice. The difficulties in making comparisons, the saga of the secure units, and previous history certainly justify these doubts. For our purposes here, however, the exchange underlines again the *limits* of central influence particularly as the Secretary of State himself in his letter to MIND acknowledges the 'difficulties . . . in achieving our objectives'. [14]

Services for the Elderly [15]

The elderly make greater use of health services than other age groups, and their number is increasing. The additional demands arising from this demographic change has been recognised and due allowance has been made in annual allocations to the NHS. For example, the government accepted that much of the 1.4 per cent annual increase (in real terms) projected for hospital and community services in 1976 'will have to be devoted to those services which cater for the needs of older people'. [16] Put another way, the increasing number of elderly has been one of the most potent arguments available to the Secretary of State in the annual debate with the Treasury on allocations to the NHS.

The 'suggested' annual increase for services for the elderly was 3 per cent in the period up to 1979/80 (compared with 0.9 per cent for the acute services). The Consultative Document also suggested as priority claims on the 3 per cent, 'rapid development' of domiciliary services, 'development of acute geriatric units in general hospitals with immediate access to full diagnostic, therapeutic and rehabilitation facilities', residential accommodation and 'special in-patient and day hospital units'. Within these desiderata, specific targets were suggested, one of which was that '10 per cent of geriatric bed need . . . should be provided in general hospitals by the end of 1976/7'. These policies (most of which pre-dated 1976) were confirmed in *The Way Forward* in 1977. The fortunes of the services for the elderly are thus a very useful test of the capacity of the centre to influence local decisions. There was not only a commitment to a relatively high priority in the share-out of additional resources, but policies were specific and well established.

Developments: 1976-9. The emphasis on this policy implicitly underlined the difficulty which the centre had previously had in persuading others.

> The document also highlights . . . the pressure on services due to the rising numbers of elderly . . . It therefore suggests that unless the targets for meeting these needs are to be abandoned, there must be a deliberate decision to give them priority over the development of the general and acute hospital services.[18]

Had the sentiments been totally shared by local managers and providers the policy would, perhaps, have merited less emphasis.

The successor planning documents suggest that the re-emphasis of the priority for the services for the elderly has not had the results one would anticipate, if the centre's wishes have more potency as a result of reorganisation. For example, the expansion of community nursing services, central to the objective of 'helping old people to remain in the community for as long as possible', has not materialised on anything like the scale envisaged in 1976. In 1976/7, for example, current expenditure on hospital services *increased* by 0.5 per cent, while that on community health services *decreased* by about the same amount. Expenditure on health visiting and district nursing did, however, increase 'slightly', while spending on chiropody fell.[19] One year's experience can clearly be untypical but the Royal Commission, looking at the period 1974-7, reported no indication of an increase in staff in the community.[20] The DHSS's plea in 1979 for significant increases in secondment for health visitor and district nurse training, contained in the annual planning circular, 'if the planned national expansion of these services is to be achieved', indicate continuing difficulties.

The annual manpower counts of nursing staff underline how difficult this process is. The number of hospital nursing staff increased more rapidly than that of community based nurses, when the policies of the DHSS implied that the reverse should be the case (Table 3.1).

Table 3.1: Numbers of Hospital and Community Nursing Staff: England, 1975-7

	1975	Whole time equivalents 1977	% difference
Hospital	115,837	127,846	+ 10%
Primary Care	27,964	28,241	+ 1%

Source: DHSS statistics for September 1975 and 1977. Figures exclude administrative and unqualified staff.

This experience could well have been echoed in the case of hospital geriatric services. Brown's analysis of a series of local plans prepared in 1976/7 led him to contrast 'some vague statement agreeing in principle with the national objectives' with 'a list of developments, mostly in high-technology services which the local people had always wanted'. The arguments used by the authorities included: 'we do not accept the priority . . . We need more money . . . Give us time . . . The planning assumptions are incorrect . . . Quality is more important than quantity.'[21] In the same year (1976/7) the expenditure per geriatric case *decreased* and that per hospital delivery *increased*. In 1979 the DHSS told health authorities that 'while maintaining, again as resources allow, planned development of acute geriatric services' they 'will need to give greater weight than previous guidance suggested to the effect on general acute hospital expenditure of the growth in numbers of the elderly'.[22] The relative priority for hospital geriatric services had thus been effectively reduced.

A key element in the strategy for improving the quality of hospital geriatric care is the location of beds in the DGH with easy access to diagnostic and therapeutic facilities (and perhaps the 'prestige' of technological medicine). The DHSS suggested that 10 per cent of all geriatric beds should be in general hospitals by the end of 1976/7 and that 'there should be a continuous programme of expansion designed to bring the level up to at least 30 per cent by 1979/80'.[23] This was also to apply to teaching hospitals, which hitherto had paid little attention to geriatric medicine.

One part of the research programme in the Institute for Health Studies took us to a teaching DGH which was being developed with a view to the incorporation of modern on-site facilities for geriatrics. Although a 'one-off' incident (as all case studies are!), it did indicate how local pressures could limit the impact of quite specific policies of the DHSS. The case is discussed in Chapter 6 but it is worth anticipating some conclusions here to underline the type of obstacles that did and can beset this kind of development. The DGH was being developed in four phases. The second phase containing about 200 beds, had been purpose-built for geriatrics but was temporarily occupied by general medicine, whose accommodation had been demolished to make way for the third phase. The third phase, providing over 500 beds (in the course of completion at the time of the study), contained 90 beds provisionally earmarked for geriatric assessment. The fourth phase was still on the drawing board.

The prospects of modern facilities on a DGH site with easy access to the main diagnostic and therapeutic departments were therefore very good. Yet the initial suggestion on the definitive allocation was for no assessment beds in Phase III, with the 'spare' capacity used to centralise obstetric services. This was amended to 30 beds after local discussions and it took a determined RHA intervention, with DHSS backing, to increase it to 60. The intervention did not, however, succeed in returning Phase II to geriatrics since the cancellation of Phase IV denied general medicine facilities.

The case demonstrates the kind of local obstacles in the path of the DHSS policy of giving a higher priority to services for the elderly. While many would agree with the policy in general terms, it will nevertheless continue to cause resistance from those whose interests are adversely affected (in this case, exclusion from new accommodation). The problems arise because the interests so affected will often be those of the most prestigious providers who will have considerable influence over local operational policies. There is a mismatch between the groups the DHSS would like to advantage, and the local distribution of power.

The intervention of the RHA, backed by the DHSS, does not invalidate the argument that the centre has very limited influence over local decisions on priorities. In this case there were the special circumstances of a major capital scheme in which the approval of higher authority is required at various stages. Where developments are not of this type (possibly the majority) the primacy accorded to DHSS priorities is likely to be less.

Maternity Services

An essential part of the 1976 policy for development was a reduction in expenditure on maternity services. The number of births was falling rapidly and a cutback in spending of 2 per cent a year was suggested. This was necessary if spending on general and acute hospital services was to increase at 1.2 per cent per year – a figure which it was admitted would not permit the degree of improvement needed to meet all the pressures facing the services – *and* additional resources were to be made available to the cinderellas.[24] In a period of restricted growth for the NHS a shift in priorities (however modest) implied a reduction for some, so that others might prosper.

This element in the policy for development aroused considerable opposition, and the BMA and the Joint Consultants Committee were particularly critical.[25] Nevertheless, ministers remained publicly committed to it. The Secretary of State told representatives of the BMA council in February 1978 that he 'stood by his declared priorities', and at about the same time the Minister of Health, Mr Roland Moyle, made a public defence of 'the Government's decision to alter the balance of services within the NHS in favour of the "Cinderella" services'.[26]

The 1978 and 1979 planning circulars suggest, however, that governmental commitment was not enough. In 1978, in a view of developments 'since the publication of the previous guidelines', we are told 'the number of births fell again, but expenditure on maternity services appears not to have fallen'. The circular acknowledges the obvious when it says that this item does not 'show progress in the direction indicated by the previous guidelines'.[27] The 1979 guidelines offer a more modest target: 'expenditure on hospital obstetric services, instead of reducing as suggested in earlier guidance, should be expected roughly to maintain its level over the country as a whole'. At the same time the circular acknowledged that expenditure on general acute hospital services would have to be increased rather more quickly than originally planned.[28]

Plans and Performance in the NHS: Comment

The history of planning warns us against unrealistic expectations of
its impact on performance. Even with the more sophisticated planning
systems now available, only the very unsophisticated would expect a
striking similarity between the contents of a plan and actual performance. The difficulties inherent in planning technology (e.g. the quality
and quantity of information, problems of measurement etc.), unfore-
seeable contingencies and changes of attitude, ensure considerable
dissimilarities. Since this is the case, we have therefore to demonstrate
that the evidence of dissonance between local performance and DHSS
policy is explained (at least in part) by the inability of the centre to
get its own way when health authorities have different views about
priorities. Otherwise the material so far may be held to demonstrate
the well-established difficulties of planning, rather than the relative
strength of the various parties involved in it.

In the case of the policy on priorities for the NHS there are two
fairly obvious possible alternative explanations for the difficulties.
The first is that the slow (or non-existent) shift in local priorities is due
to extraneous factors to which health authorities have to respond:
events make policy, or at least thwart good intentions. Significant
extraneous factors may include changing patient demand (though it is
hard to see this as a major item in such a short period), unprecedented
levels of inflation, industrial disputes and wage settlements that have
changed the pattern of differentials.

The second explanation lies in the nature of the new planning
system. It could be argued that it should not be seen primarily as a
vehicle through which nationally promulgated priorities can be implemented. If it was intended only to be a means of indicating the kinds of
things health authorities should consider, evidence of dissonance could
be held to demonstrate that the locals knew better and the centre
would learn from the experience and would do better next time. We
discuss both explanations briefly to demonstrate their lack of explanatory power. We then return to the argument that the dissonance
between central strategy and local performance is a useful indicator of
the limits of central power in the NHS.

NHS Priorities: Waylaid by Extraneous Factors?

One argument advanced by senior managers and providers when faced
with this analysis has been that the continued emphasis on acute
medicine reflects consumer pressure. The providers have to respond to

the demands of patients for acute care and the numbers are said to be increasing all the time. Therefore, until this pressure is reduced it will be difficult to divert resources to services for the mentally ill and other cinderellas.

This frequently encountered response (it could almost be considered the folklore of the service) quite misconceives the dynamics of demand for health care facilities. Consumer demand finds expression only in initial contacts with the general practitioner or by attendance at an Accident and Emergency Department (the number of these actually *fell* between 1948 and 1973[29]). Subsequent decisions on referrals, further diagnosis and treatment are made by providers and it is in this *latter* sphere of activity that 'demand' has increased most markedly in recent years. While there are good reasons for this (for a fuller discussion see Chapter 5), the fact remains that they are primarily provider rather than consumer decisions. Therefore, if increasing demand is the factor that has hindered the implementation of the DHSS strategy, it mostly reflects decisions of *providers* within the service and not consumers.

Other extraneous factors have certainly made planning difficult, though whether the consequential level of uncertainty is higher than that which besets all planners is hard to say. In 1979/80, for example, plans based on assessments of likely revenue growth were undermined by late governmental decisions to require health authorities to meet a proportion of higher-than-budgeted-for pay increases and prices of materials and additional costs caused by the increase in value added tax. These decisions also caused problems for managers since it was not clear for the first half of the financial year whether the 'deficits' would be made good in 1980/1 and this was a significant factor in determining the most appropriate response. Nevertheless, there is no reason to suppose that these contingencies (and many others not mentioned) have a systematic effect on particular services. While they make planning difficult (perhaps less so than critics in the NHS would have us believe), they do not increase the prices of particular services in such a way that attempts to shift resources into, say, the services for the mentally ill and elderly, are vitiated. Unless it can be proved that the net effect of all these extraneous factors do work systematically to the advantage of some and to the disadvantage of others, they do not offer a convincing explanation of the low or non-realisation of the centre's policy on priorities.

Priorities and Performance: A Misrepresentation of the NHS Planning System?

A more substantial objection to our use of the impact of DHSS policy on priorities on local outcomes, as an indication of the limits of the power of the centre, is that we misrepresent the nature of the planning system and the policies on priorities. The simple comparison of objectives enunciated in 1976 (for consultative purposes) with outcomes suggests a view of NHS planning as a central control system. It also suggests that we see the priorities for development as essentially directive in character. While we do not hold such simplistic views, we need to demonstrate that the control function and a prescriptive element are (or were intended to be), nevertheless, significant elements in the planning system and DHSS pronouncements on priorities.

An alternative view of planning is of a social learning process, described by Brown as follows:

> Goals are elusive. The attempt to identify them sets off a discussion from which all participants learn about the changing environment and their organisation's capacity to respond to it. Planning is therefore seen as an 'incremental' process of trial and error. The process is more important than the content.[30]

The DHSS planning guide does, in fact, represent NHS planning as 'a learning process'. It contains a diagram illustrating the steps from the original definition of aims through to their reconsideration. The steps are the familiar ones of review of existing services, selection of options, implementation, and monitoring and evaluation of results.[31] The emphasis on consultation with interested parties at each step in the process and the creation of joint care planning teams can also be held to sustain this view of planning in the NHS. The changes (on emphasis and timing) in priorities discernible in the annual circulars announcing the guidelines for development are compatible with this view of how things happen. The recognition in 1979 that the growth rates for general acute hospital development would have to be somewhat higher than originally thought because of the demands made by the increasing numbers of elderly is one possible example of the learning process at work. The author(s) of the circular explains that the

> pressures have been accentuated by . . . the reduction in the number of beds for the elderly severely mentally infirm in psychiatric hospitals and the constraints on resources which have limited pro-

vision in recent years of additional places in residential homes.[32]

The change is explained by developments subsequent to the original plan. The centre learns and thus changes the aims to which it would like planners to work.

Statements on the priorities also often suggest that they are less than prescriptive. In *The Way Forward*, for example, health authorities are warned that figures are *'not specific targets* [original emphasis] to be reached by declared dates in any locality'. Later in the document they are told that 'initially a substantially more rapid increase in expenditure than implied in the consultative document . . . ' might 'perhaps' be required to promote the 'redeployment and rationalisation of acute services'.[33] The cogency of national priorities to local needs is a matter on which health authorities are expected to have views and *act* upon. The 1978 guidelines contained similar injunctions against taking the projections of expenditure and levels of service as targets and suggested that they should be regarded as 'signposts indicating the direction of change'.[34] Later in the same year the Minister of Health emphasised that guidelines on the 'best use of resources' were 'not rigid policy directives'. He went on to say that 'wide departures' could be accepted 'as long as they can be justified by identifiable local needs'.[35]

The problems inherent in planning, particularly for such a large, dispersed organisation as the NHS, also preclude too directive a stance by the centre. Brown, in a review of the 1976 Consultative Document, drew attention, for example, to the time lag before the DHSS would have access to information necessary to monitor progress. He pointed to the use of November 1974 price base which, though updated, 'excludes the effect of wage-drift and other factors during the period of lax financial control in the year after reorganisation'. Projections of expenditure for the different programmes in the health budget, there-fore, started from a less than secure base. He also quoted the lower than expected growth in the number of consultant posts and the creation of three times as many junior posts between 1974 and 1976 as the kind of development of which the central authority needed early warning. Otherwise action to avoid a re-run of the emigration of 'frustrated registrars' in the mid-1960s could be unduly delayed.[36] The system of annual counts for staff in post also delays the recognition of changing trends in recruitment and makes manpower planning difficult.

If this brief summary describes the *predominant* nature of NHS planning, then the use of the comparison of plans and performance as an indication of the limits of central power would clearly be unfair. The alternative view would explain change or lack of progress in terms of ignorance which experience had begun to rectify. It would further hold that different parties to the process had not necessarily disagreed about the aims, but the debate had convinced the participants of the most appropriate ways of realising them. While there is some merit in this view, it glosses over the evidence of deep divisions of opinion about the priority that should be accorded to different programmes and the commitment of the centre to its announced priorities. Another plausible reason for the slow or non-realisation of the centre's aims remains, therefore, local disagreement with those aims and power to give effect to dissent.

NHS Priorities: Waylaid by Central Weakness?

In the NHS there are different views and interests, and these influence (perhaps determine) the aims of the health authorities and the service as a whole (and thus the effective priorities). It was always very unlikely, for example, that personnel in the acute sector of medicine would share the commitment of the DHSS to the cinderella specialities, particularly if their own services were to be disadvantaged in the share-out of growth monies. If there is any doubt about this very obvious observation, it will be quickly dispelled by a brief perusal of the response of the BMA and the Joint Consultants Committee to DHSS priorities to which we referred earlier.

It was always likely, too, that these groups would have a considerable influence on the content of local plans prepared by health authorities. Certainly this was a point they took up strongly in their comments on the 1976 Consultative Document. Of the comments made (summarised in Appendix I of *The Way Forward*), the DHSS recognised that it was the proposals for the general and acute hospital services which gave rise to the greatest concern. These doubts were also reflected in the strategic plans prepared in 1977. Nevertheless, the Secretary of State reported 'little criticism of the long term aims' but acknowledged that there was 'considerable doubt as to whether it is practicable to achieve them within the suggested time scale'.

This suggests that the differences centred on the pace of change rather than its direction. However, the plans seen as part of our research projects did not allocate priorities clearly between programmes and it is this process that will give rise to the conflict. Until effective choices are made, it will not be clear whether local decisions are consistent with central priorities. Even though plans were relatively unspecific in this area of choice, the DHSS analysis of plans revealed 'departures from national policies and priorities', and one of the 'reasons for divergence' noted was 'fundamental disagreement' with national policy. Together with the earlier analysis of the indications of the fortunes of services for the mentally ill, the elderly and obstetrics, this suggests that the disagreements extend beyond the means to the ends themselves.

This would certainly seem the case with the proposal to reduce spending on maternity services (though not in line with fall in numbers of babies born). In 1978 and 1979 the Secretary of State and DHSS were subjected to considerable pressure by professional interests and groups such as the Spastic Society to improve maternity services. The campaign of the latter — 'Save a Baby' — was an extensive one, reinforced by the slow fall in the perinatal mortality rate in the UK. The change in tone in proposals for maternity services clearly owes something to this pressure as well as the lukewarm response of health authorities to the DHSS line.

Indications of deep disagreements about ends (more evident in practice than in rhetoric) does not, however, sustain our view that the slow or non-realisation of DHSS priorities is a good indication of the limits of central power. We also have to be sure that the centre was very committed to a change in the balance and tried to realise it in the period under review, particularly where there was local dissent. The depth of commitment to the policy on priorities is indicated by the status accorded to it in the 1976 Consultative Document. It was more than a 'guideline' which prompted health authorities to consider their own standard of provision against a national or regional standard or average. Without a deliberate decision to give the cinderellas priority over acute services, the targets for meeting unsatisfied need for the mentally ill and handicapped, and for dealing with the growing numbers of elderly, would have to be abandoned. The subsequent re-commitments by ministers to this strategy make it doubly clear that the policy was clearly more than a forecast or an indication of what the centre would like to happen: the centre *intended* the change to happen.

This view of the planning process suggests that modifications of projected growth rates in favour of general and acute hospital services are partly explained by local recalcitrance.

Many RHAs have reported in their strategic plans that it will not be possible to make substantial progress in redeploying resources for a number of years . . .

Authorities whose plans assume that they can make little progress . . . should identify in their plans:

a. the circumstances which restrict progress;

b. the specific steps they propose to modify these circumstances;

c. the proposed timing of these steps and the scope each will give to enable faster progress . . . [37]

This request could, of course, be held to be consistent with the notion of planning as a learning process in which the central agents want to inform themselves of the difficulties and talk through the problems with local managers. The tone of the passage is, however, equally suggestive of planning as a central control mechanism. The agents are being recalcitrant, therefore check up on the reasons given for the difficulties and get them to move a little more quickly. It would be hard to convince anyone in the NHS that the second element was not a significant feature in the planning system, particularly given the need to obtain the approval of higher authority to plans.

The evidence of disagreement with the policy on priorities, the commitment of the central authorities to them and the elements of control in the planning system are sufficient to make our point. The limited power of the centre to effect change in the NHS explains, at least in part, the modifications in the policy itself and the slow or non-implementation of it by health authorities.

The Power of the Centre in the NHS: How Extensive Is It?

The power of the centre to effect change is limited even when only a modest change in emphasis is envisaged. If the 'illustrative projections' made in 1978 were achieved in practice, the share of the revenue budget absorbed by general, acute hospital and maternity services would have to be reduced by only about one per cent over the period 1976/7 to 1981/2. At the same time, the share taken by services for the elderly and physically handicapped would have to rise by just over half of one per cent. The difficulties in implementation can hardly be ascribed to radical change.

Agreement with the policy *in practice* does not, however, seem to have been readily forthcoming in spite of the limited nature of the change it implied. The largely covert disagreement can be (partly) explained by differences in ideology and the disadvantaging of strong local interests, in spite of the reported general agreement with the objectives of the policy. It is the fact of disagreement about aims that makes this exercise an indicative test of the limits of the power of the centre in the NHS. The outcome of a disagreement tells us a lot about whose will has prevailed. The outcomes also indicate the extent of the writ (more or less, rather than all or nothing) of parties to the process.

The centre is stronger when opposition is overt. A statement that an authority was not going to implement a central policy because it disagreed with it, invites retribution. Retribution is seen as legitimate because the local agency has challenged the formal position of the centre as enshrined in legislation and custom. However, this response is exceptional.

The differing natures of central initiatives (policies, priorities, norms, guidelines, exhortations etc.) coupled with the fact that they often (inevitably) contain competing claims, offer scope for different local interpretations for which there will be some authority. Opposition to the centre's aims is much more likely to manifest itself in assertions about their local inapplicability and inappropriate timing.

The centre has some power, however, with which to try and assert the primacy of its own aims even when the non-compliance is couched in terms of difficulties about means rather than differences about ends. The true nature of the local objection will often be obscured, but the procedure for monitoring and approval of plans by the higher authority does offer some opportunity of finding out. To date, both procedures are in their infancy and the abbreviated deadlines for the submission of the first sets of plans compounded the problem. However, it will be recalled that the emphasis (at least in the planning manual) was on disapproving things that were plainly wrong rather than positive approval of the contents of plans. Considerable scope for local 'inter-pretation' will therefore remain.

The integrative, comprehensive nature of planning, however, does effectively limit the control of the hierarchal authority. All the assumptions cannot be checked. In contrast, the *specifity* of major capital schemes makes the procedures for DHSS approval at particular stages in the planning process viable. Similarly, the developing machinery for medical manpower planning, in which a central com-mittee decides which additional senior posts should be established, deals with a finite commodity — doctors. In other areas of activity such as the interpretation of Whitley Council Circulars, where there is also considerable centralisation of decision-making, the issues are specific ones. The range of issues in a local plan precludes similar detailed controls (even if they were desirable, which they are not).

These specific controls are essentially negative in character. The centre can impose 'norms' in specific areas of activity (e.g. number of hospital beds) and ensure that local plans do not exceed them and respond to requests and questions generated by health authorities by giving or withholding approval. The centre has strong *negative* power in the areas where it is practicable and acceptable to have it.

There had been attempts before 1974 to *promote* a particular pattern of development, most notably in the Hospital Plan in the 1960s. The relationship between the central department and health authorities nevertheless remained essentially non-directional. The new planning system, which followed the development of the DHSS's own planning capacity from the early 1970s, thus represents a change of direction. The emphasis is changed from special, viable controls (and exhortations) to involvement in local thinking through the provision of material on which to base plans, and the subsequent dialogue. It can be represented as an attempt to create positive powers for the centre to supplement the negative ones that it had long possessed.

The material points to a continuing inability to promote the type of development the centre wants to see in spite of these changes. The DHSS's attempt to create a 'positive power' base has thus far met with little success. While we need only to demonstrate the very real limits to DHSS power to substantiate our argument that students of the NHS should pay more attention to the internal dynamics of health authorities, it is important to know whether central weakness is a transient condition. If it is, the position might change and our argument would become increasingly invalid with the passage of time.

Are the reasons for the slow or non-compliance of health authorities transient factors or are they rooted in the nature of authority in the NHS? The answers point more to the latter explanation than the former. It is true that the primacy of the centre is formally recognised and that one requisite of central control exists: the chain of communication down from the policy-makers (in theory) to those who implement it, is clear and unambiguous. However, the 'messages' transmitted through this channel are not so clear. We have already remarked on the sometimes (inevitable) competing considerations in the messages and this is compounded by the differing statuses accorded to them. Hard and fast rules of universal applicability are inappropriate given the range of local activities, unacceptable in a service in which so much autonomy is accorded to the doctors and impossible with the present technology for information-gathering in the NHS. Messages from the centre will therefore remain unclear and local (re)interpretation of its aims will persist.

Another possible reason for the comparative weakness of the centre in this area of activity is the 'image' of the central policy-maker. The message may be received and understood locally but the weight attached to it could be affected by the generally low opinion of departmental officers and politicians. The feeling that administrative medical staff are failed doctors is a frequently expressed one and the general opinion of central competence is not high. The undercurrent of feeling for a commission for the NHS owes something to these views. Whether these views are well founded (probably not) is not the point. Their existence lessens the importance attached to the messages from the centre particularly when they can be represented as adversely affecting strong local interests.

The central messages have to compete with those from other interests in the local decision-making process. Even if their salience is not discounted by the status factor, the lack of sanctions will again serve to diminish the importance attached to them in a situation where there are competing considerations. The only real sanction is dismissal of members or the chairman of the authority and this can hardly be used in a vicarious way. It is a sanction for a specific misdemeanor by a particular authority. It is worth contrasting this situation with the response of health authorities to adverse comments on local training facilities by such bodies as the General Nursing Council and the various Royal Colleges of Medicine. Action is usually prompt to ensure the retention of much valued training status. The combination of comment by bodies whose opinion is highly regarded by local providers and managers *and* potential sanctions ensures that the recommendations are accorded a high priority in the face of competing pressures.

This line of argument suggests that the comparative weakness of the centre, when it tries to act positively, is not transient. The factors that have, for example, blocked the centre's policy of a higher priority for the cinderella specialties have persisted since reorganisation and will continue to inhabit the NHS for years to come. The obstacle is the predominant ideology in the NHS which the centre does not control. While it employs 'experts' to define needs, the definitions may not be accepted by medical practitioners either for groups or individual patients. It is particularly clear in the case of the proposals for maternity services that these were not consistent with the ideology of the medical profession in particular (or more properly the most powerful groups within it), and policies had to be changed.

Final Comment

We have focused on divergences, or indications of them, from national priorities since our purpose is to demonstrate the limits of central power. It is, however, important to put these divergences into perspective. The Royal Commission on the NHS, in its review of the planning system, found that the pattern of expenditure by health authorities has been broadly consistent with the current DHSS priorities though stressing that too much weight should not be attached to the figures on which the judgement was based.[38]

This is not surprising because there are large areas of agreement about what the NHS is about. However, agreement does not equate with central power, particularly as we see the predominant ideology set by practitioners rather than politicians and civil servants. The test of the extent of power is the areas of disagreement and whose will prevails in these circumstances. Our analysis suggests that it is unlikely to be that of the centre when it is trying to promote change. An essential part of the dynamic of change is the local agency and its providers. A proper understanding of the development of health services in the United Kingdom will, therefore, continue to require an appreciation of the dynamics of decision-making *within* health agencies. The 'centralist perspectives' described in the previous chapter have discouraged systematic enquiry of this type and in so doing have long masked the very real limits of the centre's power to promote a different pattern of development in the NHS.

Notes

1. R. Klein, 'The Corporate State, the Health Service and the Professions', *New Universities Quarterly*, vol. 31, no. 2 (1977), p. 163.

2. R.G.S. Brown, 'Accountability and Control in the National Health Service', *Health and Social Service Journal* (28 October 1977).

3. R. Stewart and J. Sleeman, 'Continuously Under Review', *Occasional Papers on Social Administration*, no. 20 (G. Bell & Sons, London, 1967).

4. R. Crossman, *The Diaries of a Cabinet Minister, Vol. 3* (Hamish Hamilton & Jonathan Cape, London, 1977), p. 456.

5. DHSS, *The Future Structure of the National Health Service* (HMSO, London, 1970), para. 6.

6. DHSS, *Priorities for Health and Social Services in England*, Consultative Document (HMSO, London, 1976).

7. DHSS, *The National Health Service Planning System* (HMSO, London, 1972), para. 1.11.

8. R. Klein, 'Policy Problems and Policy Perception in the National Health Service', *Policy and Politics*, vol. 2, no. 3 (1973), pp. 219-36.

9. Crossman, *Diaries, Vol. 3*, p. 466.

10. Confederation of Health Service Employees, *Secure Treatment Units* (1979).

11. DHSS Circular HC (79) 9, April 1979.

12. DHSS, *The Way Forward* (HMSO, London, 1977).

13. DHSS Circular HC(78) 12, March 1978.

14. DHSS, 'Priorities Spending Heading in the Right Direction', Press Release, no. 78/92, 20 March 1978.

15. This section owes much to a paper prepared by R.G.S. Brown, *Health Planning Reform in the United Kingdom* (International Institute of Administrative Services, Tunisia, 1978).

16. *Public Expenditure to 1979-80*, Cmnd. 6393 (HMSO, London, 1976), p. 94.

17. DHSS, *Priorities*, section V.

18. Ibid., para. 11.

19. DHSS Circular HC(78)12, para. 4.4.

20. Royal Commission on the National Health Service, *Report*, Cmnd. 7615 (HMSO, London, 1979), para. 6.30.

21. Brown, *Health Planning Reform*, pp. 14-15.

22. DHSS Circular HC(79)9, para. 1.6.

23. DHSS, *Priorities*, para. 5.23.

24. Ibid., p. 23.

25. See, for example, the exchange of letters on *The Way Forward* between the Council of the British Medical Association and the Secretary of State. The full text of the latter's reply was published in a DHSS Press Release, no. 78/56.

26. DHSS Press Release, no. 76/62, 22 February 1978.

27. DHSS Circular HC(78)12, para. 1.3.

28. DHSS Circular HC(79)9, paras. 1.3 and 1.8

29. R. Klein, *Inflation and Priorities* (Centre for the Studies in Social Policy, 1975), p. 93. The number of attendances at hospital accident and emergency services did, in fact, increase but by less than the fall in GP/patient contacts.

30. Brown, *Health Planning Reform*, p. 17.

31. DHSS, *Planning Guide*, figure 3.

32. DHSS Circular HC(79)9, para. 1.6.

33. DHSS, *The Way Forward*, paras. 1.5. and 3.6.

34. DHSS Circular HC(78)12, para. 1.4.

35. DHSS Press Release, no. 78/397, 29 October 1978.

36. R.G.S. Brown, 'Priorities for Health and Personal Social Services in England', mimeo, Institute for Health Studies, University of Hull, 1976.

37. DHSS Circular HC(78)12, paras. 1.5. and 1.6.

38. Royal Commission on the NHS, *Report*, para. 55.

4 INSIDE HEALTH AUTHORITIES

We now turn the spotlight onto the health authorities themselves. In the previous chapter we argued that authorities have an important impact on the pace and pattern of development and can act as barriers to central initiatives. There was, however, no differentiation between authorities and the various groups which compose them. Disaggregation is the essential first step to a better understanding of the development of the services. At present these internal dynamics largely remain — to use an analogy from elsewhere — the 'black box' of the NHS.

In this chapter we discuss some ingredients that determine the nature of a health authority. The underlying assumption is, of course, that the different natures of health authorities will manifest themselves in different views on how things should be done (process) and the distribution of resources. Many ingredients are common to all and the nature of a particular health authority is the product of different mixes. The identification of these different ingredients, therefore, not only allows us to understand more about the nature of one health authority but also facilitates comparisons with others. Another gain may be wiser change strategies for the service as a whole, if the relative strength and interactions of particular ingredients in the nature of health authorities can be better understood than they are at present.

The immediate need is therefore for concepts that identify the essential ingredients in a local situation *and* provide a basis for comparisons with experience elsewhere. They also have to be applicable to local agencies with a somewhat different form to the present health authorities. Clearly, the formal arrangements will change over time and the concepts have to be sufficiently robust to encompass more than one set of them. Would-be analysts of health agencies, however, are embarrassed by the range of choice. There are many different ways of studying organisations and each has prestigious and formidable protagonists. As yet, there is no synthesis of the concepts of the formal structuralists, systems, contingency or action theorists (of various types) or psychologists (and others) in sight.

We propose to bypass this voluminous debate (no doubt to the heartfelt relief of our readers). The general framework we have adopted in this chapter is a systems one but we are more eclectic in our later choice of concepts to describe the ingredients that might determine the

nature of individual health authorities. We begin by looking at the
formal arrangements devised by the architects of the reorganised NHS,
on the basis that they have some influence on what actually happens.
It is also used as a starting point to identify behaviour which the formal
arrangements do *not* explain, and particularly local variations in
behaviour. We draw on work by Stanyer on local authorities as a way
of explaining these.[1] The way is then open in subsequent chapters to
expand our appreciation of the local health agency further by using
other concepts to describe and explain the inexplicable.

We are not helped in our task by the paucity of studies on health
agencies in the NHS (explained, perhaps, by the dominance of the
centralist perspectives outlined in Chapter 2). In the professional
journals there are many personal accounts of how policies emerged,
changes effected or disasters avoided, but these mostly lack a framework from which generalisations can be made. Where possible, we
continue therefore to use our own empirical material in spite of some
limitations. It offers a more consistent base on which to open the
debate on the nature of the agencies responsible for the local provision
of health services.

Health Authorities: The Formal Arrangements

One (long-standing) perspective on organisations is provided by the
formal structuralists. As their name suggests, they focus on the formal
arrangements within an organisation without claiming that these provide
the whole story of what goes on. Their concepts are familiar to anyone
with the briefest acquaintance with literature on management: division
of labour, specialisation, authority, chain of command, lines of responsibility and control, and line and functional management have become
part of the everyday language of practitioners and theorists.[2]

The concepts are intended to be more than *descriptive*. They are
held to have *explanatory* power — problem X is caused by the inadequate formal arrangements, say, for the division of labour — and are
offered as *prescriptions* for action. The differing natures of the concepts
can, therefore, give rise to confusion, particularly when it is not clear
whether they are being used to describe what *is* happening or what
should be happening. In the case of the blueprints for the reorganised
NHS, they were essentially prescriptive, and this should be constantly
borne in mind when we use the organising concepts to try and understand what *is* happening in health authorities. The architects of the

formal arrangements would not have expected them to be universally accepted and applied. Nevertheless, they provide the framework in which health authorities work and thus offer a useful starting point.

The central element in the formal arrangements is, of course, the National Health Service Reorganisation Act 1973 which set out the broad outlines of the responsibilities and powers of the Secretary of State and the arrangements for 'local administration'. The (in)famous Grey Book, published in the previous year, had indicated the kind of flesh that would clothe the bones outlined in the legislation. The report represented the work of a Management Study Committee consisting of representatives of the DHSS and senior personnel from the NHS, and informed by a study group that 'had the assistance of management consultants from McKinsey and Co. Inc. and of the Health Services Organisation Research Unit of Brunel University under Professor Jacques'.[3]

It will be recalled that the essence (it is not our intention to describe the detail) of the new formal arrangements was claimed to be

the emphasis . . . [placed] on effective management . . . It underlies the document's proposals for strengthening the regional organisation in relation to the service as a whole, and in drawing clear lines of responsibility and accountability throughout the levels of authority.[4]

In Chapter 2 we recounted the development of this kind of thinking in the NHS in the 1960s. The 1974 changes can be seen as its logical extension. Work study, organisation and method teams, operational research and incentive bonus schemes were already familiar facets of the NHS scene and the philosophy had also occasioned redesigns of appropriate structures for the management of particular groups of staff. The prime example (to which we referred earlier) was the nursing service with a new three-tiered hierarchy described in terms familiar to managers in the private sector:

Those who decide policy, the most senior officers, we propose to call *top management*, those who programme policy *middle management* and those who control the execution *first-line management*.[5]

The arrangements for the management of the reorganised NHS developed this theme, with a considerable emphasis on clarification of roles, responsibilities, lines of accountability and the nature of authority inherent in particular positions. The arrangements for health authority members are a good illustration of the impact of this kind of thinking. In the legislation the managerial and representative roles were separated with the latter going to the newly created Community Health Councils (CHCs). This would help to avoid, according to the government, 'the dangerous confusion between management on the one hand and the community's reaction to management on the other'. The health authority members were given management responsibilities that focused on policy-making and control of performance with executive responsibilities firmly delegated to officers. Members were accordingly to be chosen for their personal abilities rather than the representation of a constituency. The line of accountability from the periphery to the centre was to run through the health authorities themselves.[6]

The nurses, administrators, finance officers, community physicians, works staff and some paramedical personnel were organised in familiar pyramid structures with roles, responsibilities and lines of accountability similarly defined. The senior administrator, finance officer, nurse and community physician came together to form officer teams at district, area and regional levels. They were joined at district level (or area level in AHAs without separate districts) by two clinician representatives, one of whom was a consultant and the other a general practitioner in a management team, and at region by the works officer.

The management blueprints did more than specify the composition of the teams. They also had things to say about the methods of working. The notion of a chief executive officer was rejected and all team members were to have equal status. Decisions were to be based on the consensus of members, each of whom has a veto. Teams were, however, left to decide for themselves on arrangements for chairmen and precise frequency of meetings. Their formal place in the overall scheme of things was, however, made crystal clear. Teams were to be collectively accountable to their respective health authorities.

Another significant theme in the new formal arrangements was the need for collaboration between professions. Multi-disciplinary management teams were only one manifestation, and the provisions for participation by different professions were much more extensive than this. The involvement of clinicians in hospital management was, of course, already well established. It was based in most hospital groups on 'cogwheel divisions' of associated specialists (e.g. surgeons) whose representatives constituted a medical executive committee. Now the Grey Book suggested the addition of a new district committee composed of representatives of clinicians, general practitioners and community health staff. While the arrangements for other groups were less elaborate they nevertheless afforded staff the chance of participation. There was provision, for example, for the creation of area advisory committees composed of a particular professional group (e.g. nurses, dentists). The extensive provisions for participation justified by the need for collaboration in a complex service was presented as a gain from reorganisation.[7]

The planning system (described in Chapter 3) detailed the processes that would animate the new management structure, in which the provisions for professional participation were so important. The total package was intended to change the *nature* of local administration in the NHS. It was intended to enhance the importance attached to decision-making based first on the identification of ends (defined variously as needs, objectives, aims), second on the choice of most appropriate means and subsequently on monitoring and review of progress. The 'coherence' of the management arrangements would ensure that these tasks would take place at the most appropriate part of the structure and overall consistency maintained. The influence of these arrangements on local systems was not supposed to be confined, however, to process and location of responsibilities. The changes were also intended to increase the importance attached to the values of economy and efficiency in the management of the NHS.

The many shorthands to describe the kind of system outlined here include 'scientific management', and this is the phrase we shall subsequently use.

The Nature of Health Authorities: How Significant are the 'Scientific Management' Arrangements?

We said earlier that these blueprints for NHS management were prescriptive: they were intended to show the way. Some elements were, of course, more directive than others. The size of health authority, the establishment of CHCs and the advisory machinery for professional groups, the composition and method of working of management teams and the creation of particular posts, were all issues on which there was no local choice. To that extent the formal arrangements do describe *one* aspect of the nature of authorities and this is why they provide an obvious and useful starting point for our analysis of local health agencies. The blueprints have useful things to tell us because they provide us with the framework in which local providers, managers and members have to work.

The difference between what the formal arrangements of an organ-

isation suggest *should* happen and what actually *does* happen, is now a
well-established fact and there is no need to argue it here. All we need
to register at this stage in the argument is the obvious point that other
factors also determine the nature of local health agencies. A prerequisite of a study of local agencies is the identification of these other
factors. Once these are established the way is then open for an evaluation of the relative influence of the formal arrangements and the other
factors in the determination of the nature of health authorities both in
general and in particular.

Differences between and within authorities are one indication of
the existence and type of other factors that contribute to the nature
of particular health authorities. By definition, management arrangements common to all authorities cannot explain very readily differences between them. An exception is the variations at clinical level.
These are explained by the general phenomenon of clinical autonomy,
which has considerable impact on the pattern of local activity. For
example, differences in the lengths of stay for essentially similar conditions are well known and have drawn frequent comment from the
DHSS. In the first consultative document on priorities it was pointed
out to health authorities that 'if the average length of stay could be
reduced to the present median in areas where it is above it, there would
be a potential annual saving of the order of £26 million in "hotel"
costs'.[8] There is also the expected differences in the incidence of
particular procedures. The rates for hip replacement surgery, for
example, may vary considerably between regions and the variation is
not explained by different levels of resources. Liverpool region is, by
British standards, well endowed; Trent is universally acknowledged to
be very deprived. Yet the rates for the procedure in *both* regions is well
below the national average.[9] Variations in prescribing habits and rates
for abortions are also well-established facts.

All variations are not, however, explained by clinical freedom, or by
the legacies of the pre-1948 period. Local appreciation of priorities
have and do play a part in shaping developments. For example, in the
pre-reorganisation hospital services, doctors in Exeter and Stoke-on-
Trent promoted centres for postgraduate medical education centres.
The Chief Medical Officer to the department at the time has underlined just how much of a local initiative this was:

I cannot over-emphasise the importance of the spontaneous nature
of this development within the profession itself. It did not arise from
the prompting of the central department, however much it may have

been assisted from central funds . . .[10]

In the sphere of planning there have been marked differences between health authorities. Some failed to submit plans and those that did adopted different modes of presentation and approaches to the task. There were also obvious deviations from the spirit (and letter) of the policy on priorities. We have identified a similar pattern in the field of financial allocations, in spite of clearly defined policies. In our case material there were also differences between two RHAs' views on current balances, treatment of RCCS (Revenue Consequences of Capital Schemes) and the proper scope for switches between capital and revenue monies. The differing fortunes of health authorities in persuading Social Service Departments to participate in jointly financed schemes are further indications of local factors at work.

This is also true in the field of personnel management. There were marked differences in the late 1960s and early 1970s in the responses of local managements to the opportunities to introduce bonus schemes to enhance the earnings of ancillary staff, in particular.[11] The varied incidence of local industrial action, even during national disputes (e.g. ancillary staff in 1979), is another of the many pointers to the significance of local factors in behaviour. A national survey of grievance and disciplinary procedures by a student in the Institute for Health Studies also revealed considerable local variations in practice.[12]

There are other areas of activity where differences between authorities, and between units of the same authority, are discernible even to the most cursory inspection. The differences reflect the nature of the authorities and units, and are unexplained by management arrangements common to all. In the case of the NHS, the obvious universal arrangement that does, as we have said, promote local difference is the guarantee of clinical autonomy to doctors. The differences in lengths of stay, the incidence of various medical procedures and the costs of prescribing are explained by this facet of the NHS. There is, however, no other obvious feature in the formal arrangements to account for the differences in innovation (e.g. postgraduate medical centres), policies for development (e.g. plans), techniques of financial management (e.g. compensation for RCCS), opportunities for enhanced earnings (e.g. bonus schemes) and relations between management and providers (e.g. industrial unrest). The explanations lie in the particular mix of factors that contribute to the nature of a local health agency (or lower-level unit).

Health Authorities: Other Influences

Stanyer has argued that local authorities have been misrepresented by portrayals of them as an extension of national government. He suggests that *each* local authority should be viewed as a miniature political system influenced by its local environment. The nature of each authority is the product of the local environment including its traditions (e.g. (non)partisanship), the local actors and internal organisation including the formal structure and processes. The particular 'mix' explains the local predispositions that inform policy. While the central ingredient of the local authority system — locally elected members — is missing in the case of the NHS, Stanyer's schema is useful because it alerts us to other obvious influences on the nature of a health authority.

The impact of the various actors are discussed in the following chapters (in a somewhat different framework) and we focus here on features of the local community that Stanyer argues will have some influence on the nature of the associated local authority. His list of environmental factors includes:

  (i)   the proximate environment, by which he means the particular location of the authority and its history;
 (ii)   the local economy;
(iii)   the local social system;
(iv)   the local political system.

The essential points for the discussion here are whether these factors filter through into the local health authority system and their relative significance *vis-à-vis* other factors. On the second point, it might be held that the absence of elected members and the consequent loss of political legitimacy by health authorities means that other factors, including the wishes of the centre, are more influential than in local government. Even if this is true (which we do not necessarily accept) it does not deny *some* significance to local environmental factors that do filter through in some way and influence the nature of the local health agency. What we need to do, therefore, is to explore each of Stanyer's environmental features briefly to see how they can have a local influence. This will be sufficient to demonstrate the value of exploring the environment of each health authority to see if it does produce a clearer view than we have at the moment of how they work in practice.

The Proximate Environment

Intuitively, the geographical location of a health authority, its hospitals,

clinics and surgeries, do seem to be likely influences on the nature of
the local system. The industrial relations atmosphere, for example,
seems on the basis of studies of authorities in the North of England, to
be less fractious in rural than in urban areas. A possible explanation
may be the different views in the local communities on the respective
roles of unions and managers. Another explanation may be the
different levels of centralisation of services in rural and urban areas.

Another aspect of location that seems a likely influence on the
nature of health authorities is the distance from London and from the
headquarters of the RHA. Certainly, health authority personnel in the
North of England often comment on the seemingly easier access of
health authorities in London and the South East to the DHSS. Again,
the extent of geographical isolation of psychiatric hospitals (another
aspect of location) has been thought to be a factor in the outmoded
practices found in some of them.

History is also likely to be a factor in spite of reorganisations that
abolish long-established local organisations. Traditions of local agencies
that might intrude into the new set-up include attitudes to management (helpful, bureaucratic etc.) based on past events. Well-developed
understandings about the pattern of services and priorities, as well as
the accepted practice associated with consultation, are other possible
examples of a historical factor at work. Health services are still often
staffed by people with long connections with particular institutions,
who can act as the organisation's memory. This is also true of members
of health authorities and CHCs, many of whom can claim long periods
of service with the predecessor authorities. In our study of reorganisation in Humberside, nine of the AHA and CHC members claimed an
experience of over 20 years of health service administration.[13]

Reorganisations do not immediately change the expectations of consumers. For example, the tradition of seeking primary medical care in the
accident and emergency department is more persistent in some areas than
in others. One obvious explanation is the original imbalance between
the differential availability of hospital casualty and general practitioner
services in city centres and leafy suburbs. On a similar tack, the traditions of the great teaching hospitals survive to remind us of the importance of history in the nature of local systems.

The Local Economy

Stanyer suggests that data on the nature of local economic activity, the
levels and distribution of wealth and income, and the state of employment provide an elementary base for the characterisation of the local

economy. The characterisation, once established, will then provide insights into the relations of the economic environment to the local authority. The dependency of health authorities on central allocation of funds might suggest, however, that the character of the local economy has less relevance to them than to local government. Nevertheless, it is possible to see ways in which the local economy has *some* influence on the nature of its associated health authority.

The level of employment, for example, differs markedly throughout the country and over relatively small distances. It is generally felt that health authorities in London and the South East have more difficulty in recruiting ancillary staff than in more economically depressed areas elsewhere. If this is so, the quality as well as the quantity of staff that authorities are able to recruit for similar jobs will also differ. With the most senior posts, which have a national catchment area for recruitment, the position is often reversed. The more successful practitioners are mostly attracted to the better endowed areas of the country.

The structure of the labour market is again a factor that will obviously affect the volume, type and quality of recruits. In Humberside, for example, manpower studies suggest that the availability of female labour varies between the south bank (Scunthorpe and Grimsby) and the north bank (Hull and Beverley). The relatively low proportion of middle-class occupations in the area must also affect recruitment to white-collar occupations.[14]

Some might argue that these factors affect the input of resources (volume, type, quality) rather than the nature of the local system. Such a view would, however, be somewhat inhuman and contrary to commonsense. The type of personnel and the particular mix in an authority will have a local flavour and it will have some effect on local predispositions. For example, there are studies that have pointed to different 'orientations' of staff, and these are reflected in attitudes to jobs and the organisation. Blau and Scott, in a study of social workers in a US county welfare agency many years ago, confirmed a distinction made in earlier reports between cosmopolitan and local attitudes to employers and they were associated with different loyalties and willingness to criticise.[15] The link between local attitudes and policy-making was underlined in a study of decision-making in the Hull Corporation. The author identified the insularity of local councillors, which was also linked to the economic and social structure of the city, as one of the reasons for the decisions against fluoridisation of the water supply.

As the geographical isolation, coupled with the social immobility which is the result of its industrial base, produces an aggressive insularity, not least among councillors . . . Had fluoridation been devised in Hull it might have made more appeal to the city fathers.[16]

The Local Social System

Since similar arguments apply to the nature of the local social system, they are not elaborated here. Perhaps one observation, however, is worthy of mention. The age structure of the local population (Stanyer's classification refers to class, status and stratification) clearly affects the volume and type of demand on local services and therefore the spread of services provided. This in turn influences the range of specialist groups and their numbers. An area with a larger-than-average elderly population, for example, will employ more staff concerned with their care and perhaps a greater bargaining power for geriatricians. This facet of the social structure of the area will thus be a factor in the composition of the workforce, and through that it could also be an influence in local predispositions on policy issues.

The Local Political System

Stanyer sees the political institutions and processes as the mechanisms through which the local economic and social systems produce their effect. While the local political institutions have less effect on the health authority, they are not without power. The composition of both health authorities and CHCs are affected by them since local councils nominate members of both bodies. A change in political control also soon finds expression in a change in membership and perhaps the stance of the authority and CHC. There are also links between provider groups and local political institutions, with trade unions and the Labour Party being the most obvious example.

The impact of the local political institutions and the economic system on health authorities was brought to the attention of one of the authors in a very homely way in 1979. He had been asked to talk to members of a health authority that provided services for a large mining community. The Labour Party have been in control of the associated local authorities for so long that the area could be said to be a one-party state. The attitudes (and loyalties) of members reflected this situation, and the author was pleased to receive his cheque drawn on the local Co-operative Bank. More substantially, however, it does seem that effects of the local social systems and economy are as likely to be mediated through recruitment patterns as through local political institutions in health authorities.

Health Authorities: The Significance of Local Environmental Factors

Let us begin the discussion of the relative importance of local environmental factors on health authorities by summarising the argument in
this chapter so far. We have pointed to the obvious influence of the
formal management arrangements on the nature of a health authority.
The managerialist element in that nature will be reflected in the manner
in which decisions are made and the priority given to the values of
economy and efficiency. We went on to say that discernible differences
between and within health authorities suggested other factors at work
and we used Stanyer's schema of the types of local environmental
influence to speculate on the impact of these factors on the nature of
health authorities. The comparative insulation of health authorities
from the local political system, and particularly the absence of the
central characteristic — directly elected members — may, however, serve
to lessen the influence of these local environmental factors. This would
suggest that while the proximate environment, the local economy and
local social and political systems are factors to be taken into account,
they are not as pervasive as they are in the case of a local authority.

There are other reasons which suggest that external factors (of which
the local environment is but one source) have a muted impact on local
health agencies. The system of finance — funds provided (automatically) by the centre — stable consumer patterns of behaviour and
provider control of workload, means that health authorities are not
very dependent (in *fact* if not in theory) on external agencies for
essentials. The absence of local political control also means there is no
necessity to obtain community approval of local performance. The net
result is an agency surprisingly insulated from changes and pressures
originating in the environment of health authorities.

How do we arrive at this view? An overriding characteristic of a
health authority is the near total absence of market forces in the local
allocation of resources. The budget is to all intents and purposes fixed.
There is little to be gained, for example, from a zealous policy of maxi-
mising income from the few charges which exist. Again, competition for
patients is hardly a potent factor since the NHS, outside one or two
areas, is a monopoly: even where there is an alternative service, it is
comparatively little used.

Health authorities are also insulated from the problems of raising money, a process that has the effect of linking provider and the views of those more closely involved in the economic system. Even within central government this linkage is present since the departments have to negotiate directly with the Treasury for funds. In the case of the NHS, negotiations are with the higher tier (DMT with AHA, AHA with RHA, RHA with DHSS), none of whom have responsibilities to raising monies from taxpayers. Within the context of these relationships attention is focused on the distribution of monies, though with considerable wailing about the inadequate sums made available. Additionally, there is little variation in the monies made available and future allocations can be calculated with a considerable degree of confidence. In one case study of financial planning we compared the official guess for one AHA (i.e. the planning assumption) of what the allocation would be in the financial year beginning 18 months later and what, in fact, was received. Although the growth element was higher than forecasted, the total sum available was within 2 per cent of the planning assumption for that year. Since allocations have been inflation-proofed (though 1979/80 proved to be a marginal exception) this represents a very stable position and one in which the level of certainty is high. It is highly probable that this stability (maintained in a period of high inflation) also serves to insulate health authorities from the concerns of those in the economic system.

There is considerable local control over the volume of demand admitted into the system and the claims made on the allocation. At the moment there are only two points of access for the patient: either by approaching the GP, or by walking into the accident and emergency department. The introduction of appointment systems is an example of how demand can be contained in the field of primary medical care.[17] While consumer pressures on the accident and emergency departments cannot be so easily controlled, there are also ways to deter the casual minor injury, and the centralisation of these units will no doubt have had this effect. Beyond these points of entry, the volume of demand (e.g. for beds, out-patient appointments, diagnostic tests, various therapies including drugs) is largely determined by what the *doctor* thinks is the appropriate course of action, and the availability of facilities, including colleague time. In the absence of a market situation where doctors compete for patients, local providers are largely insulated from consumer preferences and health authorities from this aspect of their local environment.

There are other points of access for consumer views. The newest is the CHC which, by design, has no executive responsibilities. Health authorities are, however, required to consult them on plans for development and to meet them formally at least once a year. CHCs are involved in closure proposals and if they agree, there is no need to take the decision to higher authority. CHCs, arguably the most innovative aspect of the 1974 reorganisation, are composed of nominees of the associated local authorities, representatives of voluntary bodies with an interest in health and nominees of the regional health authority.

A second stream of public representation is found in health authority membership. In addition to the three professional (one consultant, one GP and one nurse) members and others appointed by the RHA, there are nominees of local councils and the latter comprise approximately one-third of the total membership of an AHA. (At the time of writing, proposals for the election of two staff representatives have not been implemented.) All members are very part-time, except the chairman (appointed by the Secretary of State) who receives a payment based on the premiss that his duties will consume two full days per week.

The impact of these public representatives on local decisions is hard to assess. Certainly there is a view among officers that members are not significant factors in the formation of local policies: one of the problems, for example, has been to find things for them to do. Some research on CHCs has taken their claims of influence at face value,[18] but in our studies they do not seem to be a major force in directing the development of the NHS. In discussions with a group of senior officers in 1978 on management issues in the NHS there were few references to either health authority members or community health councillors. Since the role of both were germane to some of the issues raised, we took the relative silence as a further indication of their low saliency.[19]

This may be because there is no conflict of interest between providers and the public interest. The comparative insignificance of private medicine in the United Kingdom would suggest a satisfied public. In 1976, for example, for every pound spent in the private sector, over £1,000 was spent on the NHS, and Odin Anderson in his assessment of health systems in the USA, UK and Sweden felt that the British public seemed the happiest with their health system.[20] Where there is little dissatisfaction among consumers and seeming agreement on the basics of the NHS, the primary role of public representatives may be more symbolic than managerial.

This is the reasoning that has led us to believe that health authorities are more insulated from changes in their local environment than are local authorities. The observation also accords with popular comments about the 'remoteness' of health authorities, though the critics mostly refer to management rather than to the providers. The accusations of remoteness may be due to this insulation, as well as other factors such as size and unfamiliarity with new institutions. Whatever the reason, the effect of the absence of control by the local political system would, on the basis of *a priori* reasoning, seem to be reinforced by the monopoly position of health authorities (a characteristic they share with local authority services), their financial structure and local provider control over the level of demand.

While it is tempting to take up a position on this issue, it would not be germane to our argument here. We are identifying factors that could influence the nature of individual health authorities and we have suggested some elements in the location, history, the local economy and social and political systems that might have that effect. The subsequent argument that the formal position of health authorities might diminish the influence of this kind of external factor on the nature of a health authority does not, however, deny it *some* significance. It does suggest, however, that local environmental factors are less pervasive than the formal management arrangements established by the centre, although this could differ between health authorities. It is possible that links with the local systems are stronger in some areas than others. The refusal of the Lambeth, Southwark and Lewisham AHA(T) to cut back its spending between 1977 and 1979 to match its allocation may owe something to this factor. Certainly to the outside observer, Labour councillors on the authority seemed to be influential in the stance of the AHA(T).

Health Authorities: The Importance of Formal Management Arrangements

The downrating (but not dismissal) of the importance of local environmental factors in the nature of a health authority might suggest that the formal management arrangements are the predominant influence. This is an argument we take up in the next two chapters when we examine actual practice against the theory of the reorganisation blueprints.

In the meantime, we are left with the evidence of differences between and within authorities that universal management arrangements cannot explain. If local environmental factors do not offer a convincing explanation, then we have to look elsewhere, if, as we argue, some of the differences reflect local preferences rooted in the nature of a particular health authority. The argument that health authorities are relatively insulated from environmental pressures directs attention to the contribution of the different groups employed, or in contact with them. The essential dynamic of health authorities comes from within, and their individual natures reflect (at least in part) the particular local mix of providers, the relationships between them and the processes by which decisions are made.

Notes

1. J. Stanyer, *Understanding Local Government* (Fontana/Collins, London, 1976). The many subsequent references to Stanyer in this chapter are not individually referenced. The relevant chapters are Chs. 1-4.

2. For an excellent summary of this approach see D.J. Murray, *Approaches to the Study of Public Administration, Part I. The Formal Structural Approach* (Open University Press, 1974).

3. DHSS, *Management Arrangements for the Reorganised National Health Service* (HMSO, London, 1972), p. 4.

4. DHSS, *National Health Service Reorganisation*, Consultative Document (HMSO, London, 1971), Foreword.

5. Ministry of Health, *Report of the Committee on Senior Nursing Staff Structure* (HMSO, London, 1976), para. 1.5 (original emphases).

6. *National Health Service Reorgansiation: England*, Cmnd. 5005 (HMSO, London, 1972).

7. Ibid., Foreword.

8. DHSS, *Priorities for Health and Social Services in England* (HMSO, London, 1976), para. 4.22.

9. R. Klein, Paper given to the IHSA Annual Conference, *Hospital and Health Services Review*, vol. 73, no. 8 (1977).

10. Sir G. Godber, "Hospital and Community: The Pattern of Medical Care', *International Hospital Federation* (September/October 1970).

11. S.C. Haywood, *Managing the Health Service* (Allen & Unwin, London, 1974), p. 139.

12. D. Wandless, *An examination of grievance and disciplinary procedures in the National Health Service* (Project Report, Institute for Health Studies, University of Hull, 1979).

13. R.G.S. Brown et al., *New Bottles: Old Wine?* (Institute for Health Studies, University of Hull, 1975), p. 27.

14. E.W. Evans, *Humberside Statistical Bulletin*, no. 1, published by the University of Hull 1974, pp. 1, 5, 8, 13, 16, 41.

15. R. Blau and R. Scott, *Formal Organisations* (Routledge & Kegan Paul, London, 1963), pp. 64-71.

16. A.P. Briers, 'The Decision Process in Local Government. A Case Study of Fluoridisation in Hull' *Public Administration*, vol. 48, no. 2 (1970), p. 154.

17. R. Klein, *Inflation and Priorities* (Centre for Studies in Social Policy, 1975), p. 93

18. R. Klein, *The Politics of Consumer Representation* (Centre for Studies in Social Policy, 1976).

19. S.C. Haywood *et al.*, *The Curate's Egg . . . Good in Parts. Senior Officer Reflections on the NHS* (Institute for Health Studies, University of Hull, 1979).
20. O.W. Anderson, *Health Care. Can There be Equity?* (John Wiley & Sons, New York, 1972).

5 THE MEMBERS AND SENIOR MANAGERS OF HEALTH AUTHORITIES

In this chapter we turn the spotlight from the influence of formal management arrangements and the local environment on the nature of health agencies to the people involved in them. The discussion focuses on the contribution of two sets of actors central to the management function, members of authorities and senior officers.

The main purpose is a comparison of the actual functions of these two groups with those outlined in the 1974 blueprints. Close similarities between the two will be taken to indicate that the underlying models of management behaviour strongly influence the nature of health authorities. They will also be taken to indicate a continuing strong influence in future types of health agency, since the stock of ideas from which organisational blueprints seem to spring assume a strong leadership role for managers. Slightly different arrangements, even those designed to facilitate local variations, are hardly likely to alter that situation very much. On the other hand, evidence of considerable differences between blueprints and reality will be taken as an indication that the managerial models of behaviour (and managers) are not — and are unlikely to be — a major influence on the nature of health authorities in the NHS.

Dissimilarities are, of course, to be expected. There is a voluminous literature on the inevitability of deviations from the formal management arrangements in practice. The comparisons must, therefore, unearth gross differences if we are to argue (as we do) for a very limited influence for the artefacts of scientific management philosophies, progressively introduced since the mid-1960s. Merely minor variations will thus suggest a strong influence. It is also important that comparisons must concern activities at the heart of the management function. It is for this reason that we concentrate on the ability of members and senior managers to *direct* the general development of services.

Top Managers as Directors of Development: the NHS Blueprints

The idea that top management sets the directions for development of an organisation is a venerable and familiar one. It is, therefore, not surprising to find it given a prominent place in the descriptions of the functions of members and senior officers in the reorganised NHS.

Health authority members were enjoined to detach themselves from issues of day-to-day management and concentrate on general policy-making and monitoring of performance. The content of these activities found specific expression in the Grey Book from which the statements on member roles in Table 5.1 are derived. These statements illustrate the different elements in the intended 'directorate' role of members.

Table 5.1: Functions of Members of Health Authorities

Decide guidelines on priorities and available resources;	Ensure that progess is being made according to agreed objectives, targets and budgets;
Review and challenge objectives, plans and budgets submitted by the ATO and DMTs;	Ensure that services are being provided with efficiency and economy;
Resolve competing claims for resources between districts;	Challenge DMTs on their performance;
Ensure that NHS services are planned and co-ordinated with those of the local authority;	Ensure that CHC recommendations are acted upon by officers.
Assess the adequacy of services through visiting;	

Source: DHSS, *Management Arrangements for the Reorganised National Health Service* (HMSO, London, 1972).

The descriptions of the roles of senior managers and management teams in the Grey Book and the DHSS manual for the planning system follow much the same line. In both, decisions that set the general directions for local development received particular emphasis. Teams are told that, along with members, they

have a special responsibility for seeing that those engaged in planning (1) thoroughly examine the significant problems and opportunities in their spheres of activity, and (2) receive guidance on resource availability so that they can plan realistically. The role . . . is essentially strategic and they should avoid involvement in details of planning at the operational level.[1]

The final responsibility for the plan, however, resides in the team who have to decide between proposals from the different planning groups.

Senior managers have no doubt that this is what they *should* be doing. In 1975 the Association of Chief Administrators of Health Authorities saw the remedy for difficulties about the 'medium and long term roles of District, Area and Regional Teams as the speedy implementation of the planning system'. When this happened, they saw themselves being 'able to devote their attentions to the tasks arising from the coincidence of tactical planning, operational responsibility, co-operation with local authorities . . .'.[2] The implication is clear that the late introduction of a system that would direct attention to broader issues had led to a neglect of such considerations by both members and officers. This view of the proper role of top managers is very close to that of Professor Elliot Jaques, whose close involvement in the discussions on the formal management arrangements for the reorganised service makes him an authority on the subject. He describes the thinking behind the management team concept in these terms:

> The function of such a team would not be to 'manage' the District. It would be accountable for keeping District services under review, proposing annual plans and budgets to the AHA, and monitoring and co-ordinating the implementation of AHA policies by all services within the District.[3]

A more recent view of the function of senior managers (in and out of team meetings) is contained in a 1977 report on the Education and Training of Senior Managers. It was the work of a committee of some eminence in management training, established by the King Edward's Hospital Fund for London. The report's analysis of the task of top management distinguishes between individual and corporate roles, with the policy-making function ascribed to the latter.

> 'At senior level, managers necessarily operate in two dimensions: the professional dimension . . . and the team or corporate dimension, in which he participates on equal terms with the other three members in arriving at a consensus on general issues of making policy, priorities or allocation of resources.[4]

The later discussion on the type of training required for senior managers fills out their concept of what top managers should do.

> In designing curricula for management courses, too, we would argue that the elements include such subjects as policy analysis, organisational analysis, personnel management, financial administration, information services and contextual studies . . .

The committee, following Katz, placed considerable stress on the development of 'conceptual' skills for people in senior positions. The conceptual skills include knowledge of the relationship of 'his part of the organisation . . . to the total organisation'; an ability to 'read' the social, economic and political environment 'within which his organisation operates; and strategic and co-ordinating skills'.[5]

This brief detour into the prescribed role for top NHS management (a term that includes members) is sufficient to demonstrate its similarity to the conventional view of what top people 'do' in organisations. It is also sufficient to demonstrate two key assumptions on which the prescription is based. These are considerable control over events (at least those amenable to action by people in the organisation) and a *decisive* voice for top management on the direction of development. These are the two 'tests' we bear in mind as we examine material on senior management activity in the NHS to establish (dis)similarities between prescription and reality.

Health Authority Members

At the time of writing, members of health authorities number about 2,000 in England and are the successors to the greater number of hospital management committee and local health authority members before 1974. The chairmen of RHAs and AHAs are directly appointed by the Secretary of State and receive an honorarium based on the premiss that their responsibilities will take up two days a week. Others are nominated by professional interests and associated local authorities, with the remainder appointed by the Secretary of State (in the case of RHAs) and the RHA (in the case of AHAs). Various interests, including health authorities themselves, are asked to suggest names.

The objective was the creation of an authority with the right knowledge and expertise to perform the detached policy-making and monitoring roles envisaged for them in the blueprints for the reorganised service. The criteria for nomination and selection was suitability for the job and *not* representative skills, and the DHSS provided a formidable

list of qualities that RHAs should look for in candidates for membership.

> To discharge these functions AHA members will need to be inter-
> ested in the health services; to identify themselves with the area
> concerned and collaborate with the local authorities in providing
> services; to have an unbiased and critical approach to problem-
> solving so that the right questions are asked when plans and policies
> are reviewed; to possess common sense and good judgement; to be
> able to provide leadership to officers without attempting to do the
> work that officers are employed to do; and to be capable of working
> well in a group so that AHAs can function effectively as corporate
> decision-making bodies.[6]

Other requirements were also mentioned, including the ability to
devote two or three days a month to the work of an AHA. The 'special
need' for younger people was also mentioned along with 'very careful
consideration' for 'any proposal to appoint members over the age of
66'. The selectors were told that they should also look for 'a wide range
of backgrounds and perspectives . . . from different parts of the area
concerned'. It was assumed that a 'narrow range of backgrounds and
geographical location' would inhibit the development of wide-ranging
perspectives considered so necessary for the policy-making tasks of
authorities.[7]

There were changes in the arrangements for members before the
blueprint was fully operational. The incoming Labour Government
(1974) under the slogan 'democratisation' increased the number of local
authority representatives to about a third of total membership. The
government, however, did not change the prescriptions about role.
Authorities were still expected to behave as a corporate body with decisions made collectively. The injunction against standing sub-committees,
since they would conflict with the requirement that decisions should be
made by all members at full (public) meetings of the authority, also
holds good.

This very brief description of the criteria for membership and
recommended methods of working should be set against the formidable
responsibilities described in the previous section. All are part of a considered package. The functions of authorities were part of an overall
blueprint: members required particular experience and expertise;
membership should therefore be based as far as possible on a selection
process informed by criteria likely to realise that experience and

expertise; and the internal mechanics of authorities were to be so ordered that the priority given to the policy-making and monitoring roles would not be submerged by other business.

The general feeling in the NHS is that members, by and large, have had little impact on the conduct of health authority affairs. This is particularly so if the criteria used are the consistent primacy of members' opinion in the event of a disagreement with officers, or hard evidence that the course of local events would have been different had there been no members of authorities. In one project members were asked whether they had made any difference to the course of local events, and, if so, to give an example. One thought for a moment and then confessed that the only example he could recall was the choice of name for the area headquarters. In contrast, the members of the Lambeth, Southwark and Lewisham AHA seem to have been in the van of resistance to central pressure to reduce expenditure to match the area's allocation, in the period up to their replacement in 1979.

The limited impact of members was something to which we drew attention in an earlier study of reorganisation of the NHS, though it was not, however, true of the chairman himself.[8] Since those early days, we have had occasion to look at the activities of members of more authorities as part of later research projects. First impressions have not been materially changed as a result. The original circular on membership had identified 'decisions on planning and resource allocation' as 'the main function of members', yet they played only a shadowy part in the budgetary process in the seven survey authorities in the period 1976-9. In that part of the study we were quite safe in accepting officer reports as statements of authority policy.[9]

Confirmation of the low saliency of members in the business of health authorities comes in the first research report of the Royal Commission on the NHS. This report was based on enquiries in a number of health authorities in 1977, and on the basis of these the authors said the impact of members on the service 'was felt to be slim'. This was the case even when 'members were felt to be generally competent, and their role to be either certain and developing'. Another observation in the same report on the lack of comment on this issue by staff, and the difficulty some respondents nearer the operational level had in recording 'any impression at all of the way in which members worked'[10] concurs with another finding of our own. In discussions with 38 senior officers in non-metropolitan health authorities in 1978 there were few references to members, although the topic was the management arrangements of the new service.[11]

While the conclusion may be obvious, it is not sufficient for our purposes to leave the argument at this point. We also need to examine whether the ineffectiveness is due to poor design or implementation (technical difficulties) or some incompatibility with the nature of the local process. If the former, that nature could still be predominantly managerial if others (particularly senior managers) who represent that system compensate for member weakness. If, however, the reason is the strength of other groups with different views on the way things should be done rather than inadequate design or implementation, member weakness is an indication that the managerial system may not be the predominant influence on the nature of health agencies in the NHS.

Why are Members so Ineffective? One simple possible explanation for this state of affairs is that there are no real choices to be made locally and therefore no issues to facilitate a distinctive contribution from members. Or put another way, choices are so obvious that every sensible officer and member must agree with them. The marginality of member activity can thus be explained not by weakness but by the absence of disagreements and alternative options.

Some very indirect support for this view comes from the diminishing concern with the consensus requirement for decisions of management teams. This might be taken to suggest few differences likely to threaten local unanimity. It is hard, however, to explain members' weakness in terms of few viable alternative options on the evidence that agreement between officers has been more readily forthcoming than some had expected. It is even harder to sustain an argument of local unanimity given the spate of industrial disputes, complaints by professionals about spending on management and the impact of priorities on different interests. We dismiss this explanation of the marginality of members without further argument, having included it only for the sake of completeness.

Another possible 'technical' reason for the failure of members is inappropriate selection, particularly since the number of local authority nominees has been increased. The selectors consequently could not 'control' the choice so readily to enable them to match personal characteristics and the theoretical requirements of the members' role. This was the tenor of some objections to the 'democratisation' proposals of Barbara Castle during her period as Secretary of State for Social Services. The objections, also recorded in the first research report of the Royal Commission, referred to the interests of councillors (constituency, political issues) allegedly inconsistent with the corporate policy-making role of health authority members.

An assessment of the adequacy of this explanation requires us to be more specific about 'appropriate' characteristics of members. The key ones are relevant *expertise* and *interest* in policy-making activities. We take indications of expertise as previous experience of the NHS, activities related to its management (e.g. accountancy) and relevant qualifications. Studies of local authority members have suggested that indications of interest in policy-making, rather than more specific issues, is more likely to be found in men than women, and in people from higher rather than lower social class backgrounds. It is women and people from manual-worker backgrounds, who when presented with the choice, are more likely to express preferences for more specific issues.[12] Authorities, therefore, composed of members with long experience of the NHS, relevant educational qualifications, disproportionately male and middle class would indicate that the selection process had worked. The 'right' kind of people had found their way into membership to make the theory of appropriate function a reality.

A study of members of two RHAs indicated that the personal requirements were in fact met, at least in those authorities.[13] An earlier study of an AHA produced much the same picture and personal observations of other authorities also points in this direction.[14] Studies of other authorities have similarly highlighted their overwhelmingly middle-class, male and elderly composition suggesting that the three authorities are unlikely to be atypical.

The two RHAs had a total of 35 members (of whom 31 participated in the enquiry). The level of expertise was indicated by the considerable experience of the NHS in their number. Less than a quarter of them were new to the service in 1974. (In the earlier study we found that nine AHA and CHC members put their experience of the NHS at over 20 years.) Another indication of relevant expertise were the qualifications of RHA members. Four had NHS professional qualifications while the same number were members of other professions. Another four gave management or business as their occupation and two said they were trade union officers. The remainder were housewives. RHA members were also extremely well endowed educationally with the majority holding university degrees and professional qualifications. All but two reported ordinary or advanced level passes in the General Certificate of Education or its equivalent.

This picture of highly qualified people with considerable experience of NHS affairs and/or relevant expertise was echoed in the composition of the AHA when one of the authors became a member. The 18-member authority contained, *inter alia*, three medical practitioners, one practising and one retired nurse, two academics with a direct interest in the NHS, two trade unionists, one of whom had been involved in hospital management for many years, and two senior managers both of whom had had previous contacts with the service. On the basis of the membership of these three authorities, it could hardly be said that the selection process had produced people without relevant knowledge.

The same could be said of the interests of members. The high proportion of people from professional and business rather than working-class backgrounds, indicated a likely interest in policy-making activities. This was reinforced by the predominance of men (31 out of 49 members) on the three authorities, if the reported preference of female councillors for case work holds true for their counterparts on health authorities. Answers to a forced choice question, based on the local councillor study, suggests a moderately close fit between personal characteristics and preference for the 'right' kind of activity prescribed for the blueprints (Table 5.2). (The fit between the official 'identikit' and theoretical function had been even closer in the earlier AHA study.)

Table 5.2: Satisfaction of RHA Members in Two English Regions

Which ONE of the following do you find most satisfying about your RHA work?	
Making broad policy decisions or preparing strategic plans	12
Making specific decisions in a particular field (e.g. nursing supplies)	6
Checking up on efficiency	1
Representing the interests of ordinary people	6
Being generally 'in on things' in the NHS	6
Total	31

Occasional incongruities between personal characteristics of these members and expected preference for general policy-making activity, are not, therefore, sufficient to explain the member's lack of impact. Broadly speaking, they are the 'right' people with the 'right' interests and it is hard to see how a more suitable group could be arranged. The reasons for the lack of impact are, therefore, not inappropriate selection. The reasons for failure lie elsewhere.

There are other possible (but less substantial) technical reasons for member impotence. One is the very part-time nature of member involvement. Health authorities meet only monthly and often for half a day or less. This level of involvement is unlikely to provide the ongoing knowledge required to make substantive contributions or provide the basis on which informed challenges can be made. The observer at meetings of the two RHAs made a special point of this constraint on members:

> Each agenda consists of between 20 and 35 items on average which must be dealt with at a monthly meeting of three to four hours duration and only a small proportion of the items can therefore be debated at any length. It is . . . important . . . that most items should be passed 'on the nod' and this increases the need for the officers to agree their recommendations . . . before they are presented to the members, especially as, unlike local authority members, little of the RHA members' work is done in committees and sub-committees.

The difficulties for members are compounded by the amount and quality of written information they must read. One author received papers weighing over 7lbs on becoming an AHA member, with a covering note saying that other documents had been excluded to save postage. They were delivered later by hand. There has also been much deserved criticism of the quality of information, particularly health service statistics. It is hard to see 'amateur' part-time members overcoming these difficulties when professionals have come to the view that 'mutually acceptable standards of performance [were] essential before the word "monitoring" could be said to have any meaning'.[15] Poor quality information, plus limited opportunities for digestion and probing, produces a situation in which a genius with appropriate expertise would find it hard to make an impact — that is, if he followed the official guidelines on member roles.

While these technical factors do restrict the effectiveness of the correctly motivated member, they do not offer a satisfactory explanation of their general lack of impact. The chairmen of authorities, for example, do make an impact in spite of the inadequate information base for decision-making. The greater investment of time clearly helps but there are also other factors. The greater degree of 'legitimacy' accorded to the chairman by officers is one. Observers at health authority meetings have commented on the frequency of occasions when officers and chairman were working together to persuade members to back them. The chairman often seemed to identify more with officers than member colleagues.

The technical explanations for member weakness are thus unconvincing. They assume that if the technical problems could be overcome — even better selection, more time, better data etc. — all would be well and the policy-making contribution would materialise. In our experience this seems implausible. This is a view formed in 1975 and subsequent research has not changed it.

For implicit in the debate about information is a game about power. Some members felt that officers had too much power, which could be curbed if members knew what they were doing. In spite of the general philosophy of openness, too, some officers were reluctant to risk interference by offering information too freely (e.g. to the CHCs). Like many technocrats, they saw lay intervention as potentially irrational and damaging.[16]

Additionally, in local government, councillor rather than officer control is not associated with the election of eggheads who promote rational analyses but with the emergence of groups with programmes. It is the strength of the group, plus the legitimacy which it is accorded by officers, that is associated with effective councillor control.[17] This seems an unlikely development in a health authority in which the chairman is not elected by the members and there are no axes around which groups could form. Yet without such a development it is hard to see health authority members increasing their effectiveness even if they enhance their expertise. Members' influence will not be increased significantly by technical changes in selection, information or even structure. It requires a different conception of role.

One obvious implication of this line of argument is that members have not been influential 'standard-bearers' for the managerialist strategy of recent years. One further implication is that the essential nature of health authority activity is *not* managerial since an essential element — the directing role of members — is absent. However, this is jumping ahead. The weakness of members could be compensated by the strength of senior managers. Their contribution could be such that the local system nevertheless remains essentially managerial in spite of the members' lack of impact.

Senior Officers in the NHS: the Harbingers of Scientific Management?

The material on members points to senior manager dominance in meetings of health authorities. It does not point necessarily, however, to similar dominance in decisions setting directions for development, since this is but one forum among many for debate, discussion and decision. An assessment of the impact of senior management, therefore, requires a look at their contribution in other settings to see whether or not they are likely to be the 'directors of development', and thus reinforce managerial models of behaviour in local decision-making.

In this section we first look at material on senior managers in multidisciplinary management teams,[18] which were accorded the status of one of the six key features of the new service in the Grey Book. While teams are only one locus of senior management activity, their importance makes them a significant pointer to the general contribution of senior managers.

The central issues remain (dis)similarities between the assumed diecting role of senior managers and actual experience. Similarities will be taken as pointers to a predominant influence for managers (and the philosophies of managerialism) in the nature of health authorities. Dissimilarities will point to a greater influence of groups with different ideologies.

Management Teams in Action. The four teams in the study (two ATOs and two DMTs) were from two multi-district English AHAs, chosen because of broad similarities in populations served. Both areas had urban nuclei with a large rural hinterland and the two DMTs were responsible for the district most distant from area headquarters. In all, 25 meetings were covered by the research team in the period April to July 1977. The description of business, based on the official papers, minutes and notes made by observers who attended the meetings, is intended to convey the 'flavour' of the teams' contribution to the management of the service. Statistics that appear from time to time should, therefore, be taken only as illustrative of broad trends and not as a precise indication of quantities.

The business of the teams fell into four broad categories, though quite clearly all shade into each other. They were:
(a) *Information*: items where the primary purpose was the transmission of information, without it being related to a particular decision.
(b) *Process*: items concerned with *how* an issue should be handled, rather than the outcome of the process.
(c) *Position-taking*: items concerned to establish the teams' view on

issues or discussions which involved other agencies, other elements within the health authority, or other health authorities.

(d) *Substantive decisions*: items which lead to specific decisions designed to affect the level of service to patients, or allocate resources to staff. This category is sub-divided (admittedly crudely) into (i) *routine* decisions in which well-established rules were applied to the issue in question; and (ii) *non-routine* decisions, in which the subject matter was less amenable to the application of general rules.

The balance between the items of business for all four teams is represented diagramatically in Figure 5.1. Differences between the teams are mentioned when appropriate in the subsequent description of types of business falling into each category.

Figure 5.1: Categorisation of Items of Business in Meetings of Four Management Teams: April-July 1977

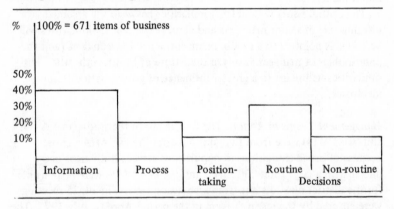

(a) *Information*. Well over a third of total items of business fell in this category in which the distinctive element is an exchange of information unrelated to an immediate decision. At its simplest, progress on an issue or development, or information on events or procedures, would be reported to the team by a particular officer; no action would be called for and the minutes would often refer to the report as 'noted'. The category also includes items which were not discussed because the information on the agenda and the acknowledgement in the minutes was sufficient for this purpose.

The types of items 'reported' in this way were very diverse. For example, at one meeting the ATO recorded the receipt of an annual report received from a DMT; noted the news from the RHA Manpower

Committee that a hospital had been approved for senior registrar training; received the news that the Consultants' Joint Medical Staffs Committee had decided to withdraw their support from District Medical Committees (composed of consultants, GPs and community medical staff) and establish their own machinery; were told that the midwifery training period was to be extended; extra funds were being made available for construction work through the Inner City Programme; the Area Medical Officer had been invited to become a member of an advisory committee concerned with training in community medicine; and the Whitley Council was debating the redesignation of medical laboratory 'technicians' as 'scientists'.

Some items did provoke discussion. The report from the RHA Manpower Committee on senior registrar posts, primarily intended for information, gave the AA the opportunity to explain to the newly appointed Treasurer the advantages of this inexpensive way of getting additional medical labour. Other exchanges of information were not directly prompted by items on the agenda. One ATO had a long, unscheduled discussion on the possible new chairman of the authority and a District Finance Officer told his DMT of a new starting date for the DGH: his wife had read the news in the local newspaper.

While about half the items in the information category were unrelated to any immediate decision, the remainder had a slightly more purposive air. An acting Area Medical Officer asked for an explanation from his fellow members on what the previous incumbent had been doing on registrar appointments; one team was alerted to possible future problems from the likely refusal of GPs to use a new health centre; and another deferred a request for finance for works and furnishing associated with the purchase of a house until the administrator had checked the procedures for house purchase in the reorganised NHS.

It would be wrong, however, to see all requests for more information as a prelude to a substantive decision. The deferments could be occasioned by the thorniness of the item. One DMT, for example, was told that one of its members had been put on an area planning team. The officer so appointed expressed unease because the decision was being made by area officers and not the DMT itself; another member felt that the selected officer was already attending too many meetings. The discussion was deferred until the next meeting because there had been 'so little notice'. The subsequent discussion at the DMT was based on a report by the appointed member, who had since attended the first meeting of the planning team. The unease about the arrangement was again manifest in the discussion but there was general consent to the proposition that agreement between officers would facilitate business because meetings of the authority itself were 'a damn waste of time as many of these members were apparently absolute fools'.

(b) *Process*. About one in five items of business was concerned with the *how* rather than the *what* of decision. There is some overlap with items included in information and position-taking categories: the differences are frequently a matter of degree rather than kind. Nevertheless, items where the central issue was process were a significant element in team business. About one-third were concerned with the allocation of responsibility for decisions to individuals or groups, usually without much or any indication of the kind of outcome which may or may not have been in the team's mind. One ATO, for example, considered a report that a list of required equipment costing £150,000 had been approved by the area's Scientific and Technical Services Committee. Items costing less than £5,000 were referred to the DMTs since items below this level were their responsibility. They were merely told that the list had been approved by the committee but the items now fell to the DMT for consideration. Other allocations concerned the responsibility for a class of items. One DMT, for example, discussed whether requests for equipment for paramedical departments should come directly to the DCP or be routed via the appropriate consultant.

Other items in the process category were concerned with the handling of an issue rather than allocation of responsibility, sometimes because the team wanted to shift the latter elsewhere. For example, one DMT had received requests for protective clothing and shoes for staff in the maintenance department. While it knew the DHSS advice on this issue and what other districts were doing, it nevertheless passed it on to the ATO on the basis that an area policy was required. Some discussions led to the matter being left to a particular officer to deal 'informally' with another agency without the team's position being particularly well defined. In one such example, a DMT wanted to go ahead with the appointment of a district physiotherapist while the ATO itself had been thinking about an appointment at area level.

(c) *Position-taking*. Items in this category (roughly one in ten) are concerned with the 'line' the team ought to take with other agencies, or whether they wished to take any line at all, on a particular issue. The other agencies included other teams, the AHA, the RHA, CHCs, the Medical Executive Committee and the Medicines Inspectorate.

This kind of activity was most pronounced in one team (an ATO) which accounted for three-quarters of such items.

The 'position-taking' related to process as much as outcome. One ATO, for example, had a long discussion on how they should present proposals for closures of maternity units to the AHA to ensure that it got the decision it wanted. The outcome was a comprehensive brief on the kind of information which should be presented and how the proposed closures of two of the units should be linked together and contained in one document.

Management Teams and Other Parts of the Health Service. One DMT used an incident to make its future position clear, *vis-à-vis* the Medical Executive Committee, on changes which led to increased expenditure. It had been told that an on-call system for operating theatre departmental assistants had been operating for some time, without the knowledge of the DMT. The team had no choice but to agree to payments for the duties already carried out, but they went on to tell the Medical Staff Committee that proposals for development should in future first be submitted to the DMT. It was up to the DMT to decide whether this kind of extension could be afforded and whether it merited priority.

(d) *Substantive Decisions.* The emphasis in these items of business is with the *what* of decision rather than *how* to handle the issue. The additional distinction between routine and non-routine is crude but necessary if we are to compare the reality with the expected role of teams in directing developments. There were a large number of items which led to decisions by teams but concerned matters for which guidelines already existed. These decisions on establishment issues included particularly those concerning study leave and expenses; approvals to small expenditures which were often minuted as approved without discussion; money for small-scale works and maintenance jobs which fell clearly within policy guidelines or were unavoidable; and ratification of decisions of others. More than three out of four of the substantive decisions were of this type.

(i) Routine Decisions. Examples included decisions on the display of 'No Smoking for Visitors' notices; on the hours of a part-time dental practitioner while another was away on maternity leave; to use the team's discretion to give a doctor a particular point on an incremental scale; and to assist with a car purchase for a member of staff. This brief

description underlines the 'low-key' nature of this kind of activity. There were a number of other decisions categorised differently but which were very similar in nature to those discussed here. For example, one DMT agreed to some compassionate leave for a member of staff, who, in the event, had already taken it. The appointment of a shop steward was also mentioned and the team reminded that the usual facilities would have to be made available. Both these items have been classified in our information category.

(ii) Non-routine Decisions. These items provide only a small fraction of team business. The comparative infrequency of non-routine *strategic* decisions is underlined by the range of items of business included in this category. Some 'financial authorisations' (a term taken from the minutes) were concerned as much with the budget heads under which expenditure fell, as the case for it. For example, one ATO decided that the costs of some expensive medical equipment should be charged against the £100,000 allocated to the Area Planning Team which was also asked to consider the case for improvements to sanitary annexes at a hospital for the mentally handicapped as a possible claim against their allocation. These decisions are included in this non-routine category of business.

In fact, debates on financial matters were never of a 'directing basic strategy' type. One ATO, for example, discussed the allocation of remaining revenue monies for the ambulance service, the Family Practitioner Committee and area headquarters. The paper prepared by the Treasurer was accepted so easily that one member remarked that the team had not really considered it. In all teams, members commented on the difficulties they had in understanding budgetary questions and what debate there was usually took place between the administrator and treasurer.

Not all non-routine items, of course, were so directly financial. Other examples included the arrangements for a seminar for new health authority members and the contribution, if any, of a nearby training institution. Another example was the response to a request from the DHSS for a review of policies for the preservation of medical records: while there were doubts about the merits of such an exercise, the team agreed to comply with the request.

Management Teams and Senior Managers: Some General Observations

The study was confined to only four of the hundreds of management teams in the NHS, and in a period that fell squarely within the learning-coping' phase following reorganisation. Subsequently, participants have argued that the now fully operational planning system may have provided the teams with somewhat different agendas for their meetings. While it is not possible 'to step in the same river twice', the material nevertheless suggests more enduring facets of teamworking which contrast with those described in the Grey Book and other official publications.

The material suggests an enormous gulf between the reality and the assumed preoccupation with strategic issues, with some attempt to proceed by way of rational analysis. Even budget allocations occasioned little debate, and in recorded exchanges on financial topics, the major participants were the administrator and the finance officer. Other team members were often quite open about the difficulty they had in comprehending financial issues, and were therefore willing to leave the decisions to colleagues. While analysis of issues is (obviously) done before meetings and in other settings, cases described elsewhere in the book do not suggest that it will inevitably follow the lines of the rational model.

The gulf also applies to the kind of issues that commanded much of the team's attention. This is not to say major issues should be their sole preoccupation, since everyone needs some light relief. Also the limited involvement of the team, in their formal corporate capacity, in the design of grand budgetary and planning strategies is understandable for another reason. Such strategies are inevitably long-drawn-out processes in which the team meeting is one theatre of operations. Since members also contribute to the deliberations in these other 'theatres', intensive re-analysis by the team would be an unprofitable activity in which to engage.

However, the balance between the items of business does suggest that the *heart* of senior managers' function lies elsewhere. The preponderance of information items in team business is a pointer to one of these other functions. The exchange of information enabled members less in touch with particular developments to be brought up to date or have the implications of a change explained to them. The minutes and agenda papers are also useful mechanisms for transmitting routine information. The learning process was particularly important for clinician members who were unfamiliar with the administrative world which provided the terminology, philosophy and business for the teams. An administrator's comment on this material underlined this point. He said that the four permanent officers had deliberately promoted discussion on items as a way of educating clinician members of the team.

However, it is the process category of business that seems to be the most distinctive contribution of the four teams to the management of services in their areas and districts. Although the proportion of items so classified was only about one-fifth of the total (and the caveat about the quantitative data is particularly relevant here), process was also a consideration present in items classified elsewhere.

The types of business included in this category represent a crucial activity in any organisation and its importance has been latterly recognised by the interest in networks and network roles. Although these terms are in danger of being devalued by their popularity and consequent imprecision in use, they convey well the flavour of a certain type of organisational activity. In their study of the planned expansion of the town of Droitwich, Friend and Spink used the concept of 'decision network' to study the interactions between various actors 'in a selected arena of decision making'. In their later studies, they came to realise how these 'personal networks, and the mutual expectations which evolve within them, can themselves provide important elements of stability and continuity when dealing with successive problem situations'.[20] Delegation of problem items to one of the team members to handle, through his well-established contacts, were pertinent examples of the same phenomenon in this study.

The impression that the essence of the senior managers' function in the NHS is the management of process rather than direction of development is further strengthened by the small number of items that did not have their origins in requests, pressures or information from other parts of the health system. There were only six issues that seemed to originate in an unprompted initiative of one of the officers. Consequently, the teams were constantly reminded of the pressures emanating from their organisational environment and their primary concern was to accommodate them (sometimes by an implicit decision not to pay too much attention) and make sure they were passed on to the appropriate organisation, committee or officer.

The objection to this line of reasoning, however, remains the jump from the particular to the general. It could be argued that strategic planning is centred in other forums to which senior managers make significant contributions. However, evidence of *activities* of senior managers elsewhere does not tell us the *nature* of their contribution. Even evidence of the existence of analyses based on rational process does not overcome this objection. Availability of data is only one factor in outcomes: how it is used depends on other factors. If the nature of team meetings is repeated in these other forums (in other

words, it is symptomatic of management and not confined to teams),
the role of senior managers will not be 'directive': it will be oriented
to process.

It could also be argued that the teams were totally unrepresentative.
There have, however, been a number of other studies which also point in
the same direction:

> We recommend that greater use be made of cost effective/
> minimisation techniques, although we recognise the general
> problem of inducing management to act on the basis of such
> studies . . . [21]

Where local problems have become serious and have led to enquiries, a
similar picture emerges. Klein, in a review of the Normansfield Report,
refers to other enquiries at Liverpool, Solihull and Rochdale, and is led
to speculate that 'avoidance of confrontations may become the
dominant philosophy'.[22] While he makes this comment in the context
of the constraints imposed on management by the principle of
consensus decision-making, our argument relates this to the nature of
NHS management generally.

The Normansfield Report underlines the problems when managers
are faced with a clear-cut crisis as they were in that unfortunate case.
The action of nursing staff to precipitate some official action on the
problems that arose with the senior consultant produced a 'casual and
inadequate response'. The enquiry commented on how matters were
allowed to 'drift' away by the Area Management Team without an
answer or investigation.[23] It is clear that the responsive nature of teams
described in our material had become totally dysfunctional in this case,
partly because leadership was not forthcoming from other parts of the
organisation. While the Normansfield situation is (we hope) very
unusual, it is germane to our theme because it again points to a non-
directive role for senior managers in the NHS. The impetus for change,
the power to block or effect it lies elsewhere and managers are essentially its facilitators.

Senior Managers and Development of Services. The secondary role of
top managers in the NHS in decisions on the direction of developments
is supported by a cursory inspection of the use of additional resources
made available to health authorities. Responsibility for direction

assumes, as we remarked earlier, the ability to control decisions on the use of resources, where there is some element of choice. This obtains when there are additional resources available for investment.

This was the situation in which health authorities found themselves in the period between 1970 and 1977. While there is some room for dispute on the size of the financial increment *above* that required to meet higher prices and salaries, there is no doubt that it was substantial. Calculations by the Office of Health Economics suggest that the increase between 1970 and 1978 was at least 28 per cent, and on another criterion was 39 per cent. This was compared with a growth of 13 per cent in the Gross National Product for the same period.[24] The increased allocations are naturally reflected in the greater number of staff employed in the NHS, and not only in the much-maligned administrative and clerical grades. The number of nurses in England, for example, increased from 270,000 to 343,000 (whole-time equivalents) between 1970 and 1977. The increase of over a quarter is more noteworthy when it is realised that the proportion of nurses in management jobs is small, and contrary to popular belief has not been increasing.[25]

However, our interest is the use of the increment to see what it tells us about the extent of management control, and for this purpose we concentrate on the hospital service, which consumes the lion's share of NHS resources. The important point to note is that the increase in the numbers of hospital staff has not been marked by an equivalent increase in the numbers of patients seen (Figure 5.2).

While some of the growth in manpower (which continued in 1977/8) was pre-empted by national decisions (e.g. shorter hours, longer holidays), the size of the increment suggests some leeway for a local say in its distribution. The small rise in in-patients treated (though there were far more day-patients) and the static number of out-patients (though there was a sizeable increase in the number of accidents and emergencies) reflects decisions not to use these additional resources to increase 'throughput'. They were clearly spent in other directions in spite of official expressions of concern, for example with waiting times for admission to hospital and out-patient appointments.

It will come as no surprise to those familiar with developments in health services to note that diagnostic and therapy departments have been a principle beneficiary of the additional resources made available to health authorities. The numbers of scientists, technicians, physiotherapists and radiographers increased significantly in this period. It also finds expression in statistics on workloads in these departments. A major use of the increment has been more diagnostic tests and

Figure 5.2: Some Hospital Statistics: England, 1971-7

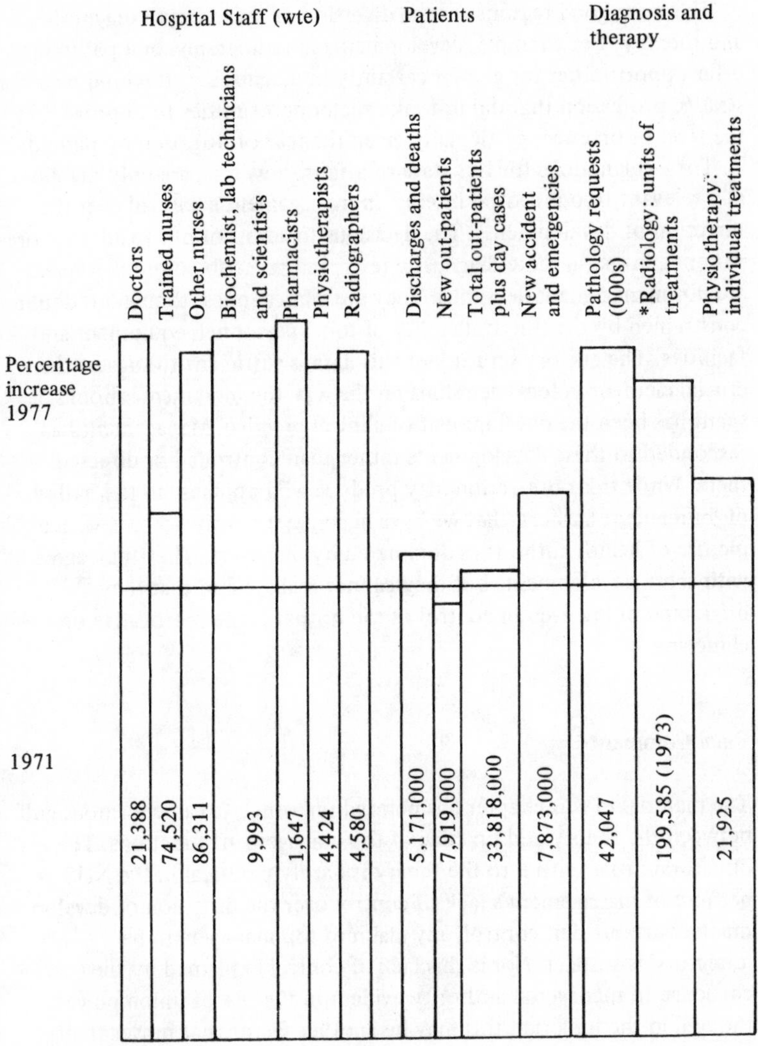

*These figures refer to 1973-7 because of a significant change in units of measurement in 1973.

Sources: DHSS, Health and Personal Social Services Statistics for England (HMSO, London); Department summaries of official returns to the DHSS. Not all figures are directly comparable because of changes in definitions. Broad trends are, however, unaffected.

therapy for a fairly static number of patients rather than the admission of more of them into the hospital system.

There are good reasons for the diversion of resources to diagnosis and therapy. For example, developments in radiography and pathology offer opportunities for greater certainty in diagnosis.[26] It would be a strange profession that did not take such opportunities to improve the level of practice, particularly given the fear of litigation by patients.

The explanations for this state of affairs, however, are only marginally relevant to our central interest in management's control over the direction of developments. The decisions to admit or not to admit more patients, invest in more diagnostic tests, and prescribe more therapies are *not* management decisions. They are clinical ones, though no doubt constrained by the (un)availability of time, personnel, equipment and facilities. The cursory scrutiny of this data is sufficient to suggest the crucial element in local decisions on the way the increments should be spent has been the development of clinical practice. Management has responded to these developments rather than controlled or directed them. While this observation may produce wild applause in the nation of 'bureaucrat-bashers' that we have become, it hardly accords with a picture of health authorities dominated by managers. They may agree with these developments but they cannot really claim that they originated or are even in control of them: that is the prerogative of clinicians.

Final Comment

The material in this chapter has pointed unerringly to an enormous gulf between the theory and practice of top management functions. The directorate role central to the theory is hardly practical in the NHS because of management's lack of control over the direction of developments: without that control, any claim of top managers to be 'directors' is suspect. Nor is this lack of control explained by the challenge to managerial authority evident in the rise of union power, though, in the long run, this may be another factor that moves their function further away from setting the directions for the organisation. In the case of managers in the NHS, their lack of control is explained by the power of providers, rooted in freedoms accorded to professionals.

The earlier material on the weakness of members and the activities of senior officers should not, therefore, be viewed as evidence of aberrations from the rightful role of top managers. It reflects the contribution that this kind of organisation needs from them. They service rather than control the decisions that effectively decide the direction of development. More importantly for our thesis, it underlines the obvious fact that the nature of health authorities is not likely to be predominantly managerial. The way local power is used, therefore, will be better understood by putting aside the managerial models of behaviour that have underpinned many of the reforms of the last two decades. Similarly, change strategies informed by the latest managerialist ideas are likely to be only marginally effective at best, and counter-productive at worst.

There are different strands to what we have called the scientific management philosophies and we need to be a little clearer about the impact of each of them. All we have done in this chapter is to demonstrate that the cornerstone of the entire package — the directing role of top management — does not seem to apply in practice. Some of the other elements might, nevertheless, have a greater impact. The three main elements in the package are:

(i) a *structure* in which responsibilities and relationships are clearly defined, usually in the context of a hierarchy;

(ii) decision-making processes informed as far as humanly possible by rational analysis, with the identification of ends prior to the choice of means; and,

(iii) pre-eminence for the values of economy and efficiency in decisions.

Clearly, the ideas on structure have taken root in the formal management arrangements for the NHS. The jargon of the management scientists is now part of everyday discussions in the service. Similarly, the ideas on process have found tangible expression in the planning system and, even before that was launched, in efforts to plan capital programmes. The need for economy and efficiency are also stressed at every opportunity by managers and clinicians alike. The adoption of the artefacts of the philosophy, however, does not necessarily mean that they determine the nature of the health agencies. The evidence we have adduced suggests that they provide the arenas and language for decision rather than dominate its substance. The evidence of the service rather than directing role for top managers, plus the suggestions of analysis that could hardly come in the 'rational' category in the descriptions of team business, points to the very limited impact of the managerial philosophies.

The elements in the philosophies cannot be very influential if they do not accord closely even with the behaviour of top managers. They are, after all, presumably the guardians and promoters of this philosophy and the growth in the number of administrators and finance officers owes a lot to the espousal of these ideas. The preoccupation of top managers with activities that cannot be understood by reference to scientific management ideologies (except perhaps merely as aberrations) also points to local systems primarily characterised by other notions. It is to the latter, and the groups which uphold them, that we must turn to understand the nature of health authorities and therefore the ways in which they are likely to use the considerable room for manoeuvre available to them. In the next chapter we discuss the impact of clinicians as the group most likely to hold different ideas about the appropriate process and values and have the power to ensure their pre-eminence in local decision-making.

Notes

1. DHSS, *The National Health Service Planning System* (HMSO, London, 1976), para. 1.4.

2. Association of Chief Administrators of Health Authorities, *A Review of the Management of the Reorganised NHS* (Report of a Working Party, 1975), para. 9.3.

3. E. Jaques (ed.), *Health Services* (Heinemann, London, 1978), p. 143.

4. King Edward's Hospital Fund for London, *The Education and Training of Senior Managers in the National Health Service* (Report of a Working Party, 1977), p. 14.

5. Ibid., p. 27.

6. DHSS Circular HRC(73)24, paras. 9 and 10.

7. Ibid.

8. R.G.S. Brown *et al.*, *New Bottles: Old Wine?* (Institute for Health Studies, University of Hull, 1975).

9. H.J. Elcock and S.C. Haywood, with T.L. Jones *Research Report on Decentralised Administration in the NHS*, for the Social Science Research Council, University of Hull, 1980.

10. Royal Commission on the National Health Service, *Research Paper*, no. 1. (HMSO, London, 1978), para. 10.13.

11. S.C. Haywood *et al.*, *The Curate's Egg . . . Good in Parts. Senior Officer Reflections on the NHS* (Institute for Health Studies, University of Hull, 1979).

12. Committee on the Management of Local Government, *Volume 2*, Ch. IV, (HMSO, London, 1967).

13. H.J. Elcock, 'Regional Government in Action', *Public Administration*, vol. 56, no. 4 (1978). The subsequent references to RHA members are also derived from this work.

14. Brown, *New Bottles*, pp. 29-30. Subsequent references to the 'earlier' study of AHA members also refer to this report.

15. King Edward's Hospital Fund for London, *Putting Meaning into Monitoring*, Report of a Conference, 1978.

16. Brown, *New Bottles*, p. 100.

17. M.J. Hill *The Sociology of Public Administration* (Weidenfeld & Nicolson, London, 1972), Ch. 11.

18. This material was published in slightly different form in Centre Eight Papers, *Health and Social Service Journal*, under the title 'Team Management in the NHS – What is it all about?' (5 October 1979).

19. DHSS, *Management Arrangements in the Reorganised NHS* (HMSO, London, 1972), para. 1.6.

20. J. Friend and P. Spink, 'Networks in Public Administration', *Linkage Three*, a publication of the Institute for Operational Research, July 1978.

21. Royal Commission on the National Health Service, *Research Paper*, no. 2 (HMSO, London, 1978), paras. B8.24 and C2.21.

22. R. Klein, 'Normansfield: Vacuum of Management in the NHS', *British Medical Journal* (23-30 November 1978).

23. *Report of the Committee of Enquiry into Normansfield Hospital*, Cmnd. 7357 (HMSO, London, 1978), p. 278.

24. Office of Health Economics, *The Cost of the NHS* (1978).

25. Royal Commission on the National Health Service, *Report*, Cmnd. 7615 (HMSO, London, 1979), para. 4.12.

26. 'New Alternatives in the NHS', Report of a Conference, *British Medical Journal* (2 November 1974), p. 277.

6 HEALTH AUTHORITIES: THE IMPACT OF MEDICAL STAFF[1]

The argument to date suggests that the formal arrangements, and particularly elements designed to promote scientific management behaviour, are not the crucial influence on the nature of health authorities. The material in the previous chapter pointed clearly to a process at variance with the official model, with a management role different to that described in most textbooks. The obvious conclusion was a continuing, decisive influence for doctors. We argue in this chapter that this influence is used in ways inconsistent with managerial models of behaviour.

The power of the medical profession in the delivery of health care is a general factor, like the formal management arrangements, that obviously has an impact on the nature of *all* health authorities. However, an accommodation between these two factors (and others such as the local environment) has to be worked out at *local* level. We therefore discuss medical power as a universal phenomenon that finds different expression in different settings. The different ways in which this and other (e.g. commitment to managerialism) phenomena are accommodated are linked with different views on the right process and priorities and, through them, to local policy stances.

While our interest is primarily the way these different factors do interact at local level, a secondary concern remains their relative general influence on local systems. It is important to sketch out the parameters within which we can expect local variations. The *general* influence of the medical profession is therefore a theme in this chapter in the context of the relative position of managers and doctors. The primary focus, however, remains the way this power finds local expression and its impact on the nature of the health authority.

The chapter begins with an outline of the general arrangements for medical involvement in local decision-making. This description and assessment of their nature provides the context for the discussion of particular cases, again mostly based on our own research programme. The chapter concludes with some generalisations on our themes of how the power of the medical profession finds local expression and its relative influence *vis-à-vis* other factors.

Medical Involvement in Health Authority Decision-making: The General Arrangements

The format for increased medical involvement in management, known popularly as the Cogwheel system, was designed by a joint working party appointed by the Minister of Health and the Joint Consultants Committee. The concern with managerial efficiency and its assumed relationship with organisational arrangements was manifest in its terms of reference: 'To consider what developments in the hospital service are desirable in order to promote improved efficiency in the organisation of medical work.'[2]

The working party produced three reports, the first outlining a more formal structure to supplement the existing advisory committees. The other two assessed the progress made in implementing the structure, and adjusted the basic model in the light of it and other managerial changes in the health service. We shall concentrate on the first and second reports and on the arrangements recommended in the Grey Book, as these provide the basic framework for medical participation in local management.

The First Cogwheel Report (1967)

The first concern of the working party was to establish the importance of management for clinicians, and their own responsibilities in this direction.

> The hospital service is the most complex, sophisticated and costly sector of the medical care services . . . Problems of management proliferate in an organisation with many branches, many functions, and many specialties . . . we believe that many clinicians fail to appreciate fully the importance of their role in management problems.

The solution was seen to be the co-option of clinicians into the management system, both to protect medical interests and promote efficiency. The report had begun by pointing to deficiencies in the present arrangements and particularly the inefficient use of beds, variation in treatment patterns and lack of co-ordination and planning. Since clinical decisions were so important, both in the use of resources and in the general administration of hospitals, it was also crucial from the managers' point of view to increase the involvement of doctors. Otherwise managerial values would continue to go unheeded.

The working party recommended a two-tiered 'managerial' structure for hospital clinicians. The first level was to be the divisions for groups of specialists utilising one DGH. The second tier, the Medical Executive Committee, was composed of representatives of the divisions whose function was to co-ordinate the activities of its constituent members with the implication that they were to exert a collective control over individual consultants and monitor resource utilisation. The functions of the Medical Executive Committee were also expressed in managerial terms.

> The executive committee and its chairman would receive and consider reports put to them by divisions, review major issues of policy and planning, and coordinate the medical activities of the hospital as a whole.

The working party recognised that the new managerial ideology would have to be introduced through the general re-education of the medical profession and specialist education for the new clinician/administrators. It recommended special training for the chairmen of Medical Executive Committees, although these posts were part time and with a limited term of office. In addition, the working party recommended the development of a new medical specialism to provide the information needed by the new divisions and medical executives about populations and needs. There were to be administrative medical officers at all levels, trained not as 'personal doctors' caring for individual patients, but as specialists in the medical care of communities. These doctors, later to emerge as DCPs, were to practise medicine in relation to populations and groups.

There are parallels between this structure and the pyramidical arrangements for other staff. The division of responsibilities between the divisions and the executive committee echoes that in the Salmon structure between the nursing officer and the chief nursing officer. Differences between the two were not, however, confined to a representative rather than a line system: the blueprints for the organisation of medical staff were not directive. The working party had concentrated on sketching in the overall framework rather than prescribing in detail:

> the radical revision of traditional methods of organising medical work in hospitals . . . must be the outcome of local consideration and conviction rather than the imposition of detailed methods

arbitrarily defined centrally.

The Second Cogwheel Report (1972)[3]

In some ways the second Cogwheel report provides the link between the first report and the structure in the reorganised NHS. It charts the progress of the Cogwheel reorganisation and points the way forward to consensus or team management, which was a central element in the 1974 formal management arrangements.

The authors of the second report were disappointed with the overall progress and the way in which the system was operating, although 48 per cent of *large* general hospital groups had adopted the full Cogwheel structure of divisions and a Medical Executive Committee. In all, of the 309 hospital groups in England and Wales on 31 March 1972, 157 (just over half) had no Cogwheel system, 30 had only divisions and 122 had the full two-tiered structure.

Problems were also reported in those groups that had implemented full or partial Cogwheel systems. In some, existing Medical Advisory Committees continued to exist without clear differentiation of function, leading to a proliferation of committees. Consultants were also unwilling to be co-opted into the managerial system, treating members of the medical executive as delegates rather than representatives or regarding the committee as advisory. In the latter case they were unwilling to allow it managerial functions, in that they did not feel bound by its decisions. Some had formalised this pattern by direct elections by all consultants to the Medical Executive Committee, turning it into an independent body rather than a second tier based on the Cogwheel divisions.

The managerial function of the Medical Executive Committee had been further 'diluted' by the short tenure of most of the chairmen, with nearly one-fifth being elected for one or two years. Since many experienced clinicians were reluctant to take on additional administrative duties, chairmen did not have the status and seniority to act as representatives for their colleagues.

The working party responded to this situation by reasserting their original ends, particularly the managerial function of the medical executive. It pointed out that the term 'medical executive' was deliberate:

The word 'executive' has the connotation of 'getting things done' and correctly describes the role that we consider the committee should play. This does not mean that it should in any sense give directions to medical staff on the discharge of their clinical duties, but that, in consultation with medical staff and others, the MEC should set and order objectives in the field of medical policy, review performance in relation to them, and work to secure their attainment by taking action within its discretions.

The working party did, however, abandon some of the means for achieving its ends. While one of their original objectives had been to formalise organisational arrangements, the emphasis in the second report changed to the underlying processes and intentions. 'The quintessence of Cogwheel is to be found as much in the attitude of mind of those who embrace change as in the structure they adopt.' The new emphasis was directed at two different situations. First, hospital groups for whom the full system was inappropriate but who could find some other method of achieving the managerial objective. Second, for groups who had adopted the forms but without the accompanying managerial process (e.g. where the medical executive functioned as advisory committee).

The emphasis in the discussion of medical management also shifted from policy-making and policy-execution to leadership.

> Prior consultations, or at least full explanation of reasons for action, is needed both to improve the quality of decisions *and to increase the likelihood of concurrence with the action that follows.* This is the hallmark of good management in any situation and places practical constraints upon the modern manager, whose position in this respect has elements in common with that of a representative leader of a group of equals who is given the power to act by his colleagues [emphasis added].

The power of the chairman of the Medical Executive Committee was also redefined and limited. He was to be more of a representative and less of an executive.

> Some decisions will require medical staff action if they are to be fully implemented and *whilst he cannot guarantee such action on the part of equal colleagues* the Cogwheel structure is available to attempt to resolve difficulties that stand in the way [emphasis added].

The second report also developed proposals to strengthen the managerial function through improved interdisciplinary co-ordination. Membership of the divisions was to be extended to include junior doctors, administrators and administrative nurses, and the chairman of the Medical Executive Committee was to be a member of an interdisciplinary management team then developing in a number of hospital groups. This management team was to form a collective chief executive implementing the policy decisions of the local health agency (Board of Governors or Hospital Management Committee). The functions of this executive were described in formal or in traditional managerial terminology.

The previous advisory committee system had informally co-opted the medical profession into the management process. The objectives of the proposals for multi-disciplinary management teams were to formalise this co-option and thereby make the medical profession accept the burdens of and responsibility for power. The working party's hope was that the medical member on the management team would act as a representative of his colleagues who, having been involved in the process, would feel bound by the decisions.

Reorganisation and the Grey Book

The idea of a general management team and the associated principle of collective responsibility or consensus management, became one of the key features of the post-1974 arrangements. The idea of a chief executive officer was rejected and a collective one – the DMT – was created instead. All team members were to participate in and conversely be bound by group decisions. Members were to have a collective responsibility.

> The DMT will be a group of equals [and] . . . brings together, to make decisions *and to share in joint responsibility*, both clinicians and officers accountable to the AHA for hierarchically-organised services [emphasis added] .[4]

The composition of the team was also designed to balance competing interests, but the presence of three medical practitioners (half the membership) might be held to be intended to give the profession the dominant voice. In other words, had the policy of co-option into the management system merged into a policy of control of it by the medical profession? The different backgrounds and interests of the three, however, made this unlikely. There is a marked difference in role between the two representative clinicians (a consultant and a GP) and the DCP who was supposed to represent the medical needs of the community. The latter is best classified with full-time members since he is a clinician turned administrator (like the nursing officer). All are responsible for their 'departments', whereas the clinicians are elected representatives of the District Medical Committee.

This district committee was intended to be the top tier of medical management by replacing the Medical Executive Committee. Unlike the latter, the new committee was to represent both hospital doctors, GPs and those engaged in public health. The chairmanship and vice-chairmanship of the committee were to be shared between hospital doctors, and both incumbents were to be the clinical members of the DMT.

This system was clearly designed to bind the medical profession even more firmly into the management process. The District Medical Committee was to have both advisory and executive roles, and the two representatives were not delegates.

> When they agree a DMT decision, they will in effect be judging that they have, or that it is reasonably likely that they will be able to obtain, the support of their colleagues.[5]

Medical Participation in Management: Comment

The structures commended by the working party on the organisation of medical work and the Grey Book have largely come to pass. There are local variations but there is still considerable similarity in the mechanisms in different AHAs for medical participation in management. Our comments on the kind of local system that the mechanisms were designed to promote are therefore based on the universal prescriptions (which may exist nowhere in pristine form).

It is clear from the foregoing description of the development of this machinery that it was intended to reinforce the primacy of managerial values, in particular the efficient deployment of labour and the use of skills. The same objectives had been present in the reports on the organisation of nursing and ancillary services,[6] but the strategy to give effect to them were different. The differences reflected variations in the traditional organisation of work — at one extreme the independent practice of the medical profession, and at the other ancillary workers whose job content was firmly determined by management and variations in the power of different groups.

The variations in power and organisation between the three groups gave rise to different strategies. Ancillary staff posed no problem since they could be (and were) directly subjected to managerial control. The strategy for nurses had to take account of some collective power and, particularly, the individual power of matrons. The latter were co-opted into the management structure as chief nursing officers and they, in turn, subjected the rest of the nursing profession to managerial control. The power of the medical profession (individually and collectively) made their incorporation more problematic. The policy of collective co-option into the managerial structure presaged less power for the administrator (particularly the group secretary as the chief executive), but in exchange the medical profession should acquire responsibility for management. The loss of power for the manager is, in theory, offset by the strengthening of the managerial function, through the co-option of groups who would otherwise oppose it.

The classic analysis of co-option is Selznick's study of the development of the Tennessee Valley Authority. He defines it in the following way: 'co-option is the process of absorbing new elements into the leadership or policy-determining structure of an organisation as a means of averting threats to its stability or existence'.[7] A similar point is made by Flanders in his analysis of industrial relations in manufacturing industry. He was acutely aware of power as a key determinant of relations, and of the ultimate significance of consensus management as a technique for co-opting leaders of the workforce into management: 'The paradox, whose truth managements have found it so difficult to accept, is that they can only regain control by sharing it.'[8]

It is important to note the different role of the managerial ideology in industrial organisations and the National Health Service. In the former, managerialism legitimises the existing distribution of power, i.e. the right of managers to manage. In the latter case it is attempting to affect a redistribution of power to administrators from front-line staff and change the nature of decision-making by making the latter managerially conscious.

While an appreciation of the strategy and mechanisms of co-option is important, the main interest for the argument here is the effect of the participative structure on the nature of health authorities. The intention is obvious and consistent with the other changes in management arrangements in the NHS. The effect of the mechanisms for co-option was intended to be supportive of the ideology of what we have called scientific management. If it has had this effect, then the nature of health authorities will be predominantly managerial — both in the way decisions are reached and the values that are given precedence, although as we noted in the previous chapter the behaviour of management in our studies was not consistent with this view.

In the next section we examine case study material on decisions in which clinicians were involved. The first study examines briefly the development (or lack of it) of the structures for medical management in two English health districts. The second concerns the allocation of beds in a DGH and to which we referred earlier (see pp. 53-4). The focus of attention is the nature of the medical contribution, and its resemblance to scientific management models of behaviour. This theme is taken up in the final section of the chapter with only brief comments at the end of the case studies themselves.

Doctors and Management in Action in the Reorganised NHS

The Cogwheel Structure in Two Small Districts[9]

The first study concerns the failure of the Cogwheel/reorganisation system for medical management in two English health districts. Both were small, with scattered services and no large scale service developments in prospect at the time of the study (1977/8). There was a consensus of opinion among administrators and clinicians in both districts that the District Medical Committee and the Cogwheel divisions (created in 1974) had failed. While the District Medical Committee continued to exist formally, the effective medical decision-making body was the Medical Executive Committee. The majority of divisions had ceased to exist.

District A. The District Medical Committee still met (once a month at lunchtime), but it was not seen by the DMT as a power to be considered or as a body that merited consultation during decision-making. When it did meet, the committee did not generate items that the three medical members could take back to their DMT. The only business came from those same three members.

The most common explanation given for its failure was the traditional antagonism between consultants and GPs. Consultants, who might conceivably feel bound by a decision made by their peers on the Medical Executive Committee, responded differently to a decision of the District Medical Committee influenced by GPs. The GPs' representative on the DMT also felt that the District Medical Committee did not fulfil any needs of his members. They had their own representation at AHA level (e.g. the Local Medical Committee and the Family Practitioner Committee) and most of the committee's business was not relevant to GPs. In common with nearly every doctor interviewed, he claimed that there were too many committees, especially considering how few administratively minded doctors there were. He did not accept the argument that every clinical decision had a managerial dimension.

The history of the Cogwheel divisions was similar. Five had been established originally but these had quickly been reduced to three. In 1975 power was formally transferred to the Medical Executive Committee from the divisions, although they could continue to meet if they so wished. By 1977 the divisions, stripped of their executive functions, met infrequently. The Division of General Medicine met once every three months; Surgery and Anaesthetics met once a year but only when there was something special to discuss; and Paediatrics and Psychiatry, amalgamated because of the importance of child psychiatry in the district, met once a month, but even this had started to drop off. The secretary (an administrator) of the latter division (the only active one left) argued that it had been a mistake to strip the divisions of their executive functions. His had provided a forum where consultants could meet with nurses, local authority social workers and psychologists. The loss of interest was blamed on the chairman for not being 'meeting minded' and on the local authority social workers for not wanting to be involved on a regular basis.

District B. In District B, the local situation was even further removed from the recommended formal arrangements. The District Medical Committee had not met for 18 months and divisions had been totally abandoned.

The consultant representative on the DMT was responsible for calling meetings as chairman of the District Medical Committee (and Medical Executive). However, he did not believe that the medical committee should exist and therefore had no intention of calling a meeting until there was in his opinion sufficient items for a reasonable agenda. He had chaired previous meetings without adequate agendas, had found them embarrassing and did not wish to repeat the experience.

He felt the GPs were responsible for the failure of the District Medical Commitee. Their independent contractor status meant that the 40 GPs in the district would not accept any six of their number as representatives. In any event, GP affairs were settled by an informal (telephone) network, and only one agenda item had ever originated from a GP, and he classified that as a moan. In the opinion of the chairman, GPs should not get involved in hospital matters. However, if they really did want to, then the weekly clinical sessions at the hospital were a more useful forum than the District Medical Committee.

The basis of the chairman's refusal to activate the committee seemed to be the traditional hostility between consultants and GPs. This hostility was phrased in terms of the superior financial position of GPs – better pay and a better tax position – and the shift in the division of labour between consultants and GPs in favour of the latter, who were said to be off-loading work on to casualty and out-patients' departments.

The vice-chairman (the DMT's GP representative) did not accept this analysis. He argued that the lack of meetings deprived the GPs of an important forum. When crises arose – as in the case of the proposed closure of a local maternity unit – the GPs had had to call a special meeting. The GPs were now organising their own district body consisting of the six GP representatives of the District Medical Committee, which he accepted was unlikely to be reconstituted. In the meantime the DMT was being used as a substitute.

In his view it was not the GPs but the consultants that were disorganised and schismatic. GPs shared the same interests – there were no specialty boundaries and the BMA had always acted as an effective political agent for them. He pointed out that GPs had always been independent contractors within the NHS and were therefore more interested in committees that would protect their interests and status. In contrast, consultants had no equivalent common interests.

At the time of the field work, the chairman's refusal to call a meeting was creating a serious problem. Since the District Medical Committee had not met for a year, the terms of office of its chairman and vice-chairman, who are also the medical practitioner representatives on the DMT, had expired. Consequently, the legality of the DMT itself had been questioned. The four permanent officers had responded by bringing pressure on the chairman to call a meeting, and trying to find sufficient business for a meeting.

The Medical Executive Committee in the absence of its chairman also engaged in a similar exercise. However, it suggested as one possible solution, the dissolution of the District Medical Committee. The discussion was only abandoned when the district administrator pointed out that since the Medical Executive Committee was, in fact, a subcommittee of the District Medical Committee, it had no power to discontinue its own parent body.

The Cogwheel divisons had been oriented towards the Medical Executive (*not* District Medical) Committee, which disbanded them at an open meeting of consultants. The initiative for the move seems to have come from the chairman, who told the research team that he had been under pressure from most of the other consultants to shut down the

divisions. Consultants saw themselves as overburdened with administrative work and felt that there were too many tiers and committees
and the divisions had been seen as the least effective.

The District Nursing Officer, who had been a member of the
Surgical/Diagnostic Division, argued that the pressure for dissolution
had come from the specialties that had only one consultant appointment in the district. There was a tendency for them to be swamped in
the multi-specialty divisions by consultants from larger specialties.
However, they gained from a Medical Executive Committee composed
of one representative from each of the districts' specialties.

With the demise of the divisions, several functions were taken over
by *ad hoc* meetings called for other purposes. For example, matters
such as appointments or holidays for physicians were discussed at the
end of weekly clinical meetings held for teaching purposes. This
meeting usually brought together some consultants, who would have
attended meetings of the Medical Division, plus junior doctors, but not
nurses. When junior doctors had indulged in 'industrial action', the consultants had used this meeting to discuss their response. The surgeons
had a similar arrangement. Some consultants questioned the efficacy of
these alternatives. For example, one argued that the utility of these
meetings for administrative purposes was limited by the attendance —
the major attenders were the junior doctors, with the majority of consultants absent unless they had a special interest in the case being presented.

Cogwheel plus Reorganisation in Action: Preliminary Comment

There have been widely reported problems with the Cogwheel structure
as developed by the formal management arrangements for the reorganised service.[10] The difficulties experienced by doctors in these two
health districts are not unusual and there is therefore, a reasonable pre-
sumption that the precipitating factors tell us something about the
general medical response to co-option into the management process.
The unique feature is the way the response manifests itself in a
particular locality.

In both cases the demise of the formal machinery suggests a dynamic
at variance with that of scientific management. The notion of hierarchy, central to the latter, is not accepted and the local medical staff
are strong enough to ensure that it is not operated. The notion of a
general interest in which the managerial values of efficiency and economy are paramount is similarly not sufficient to capture the attention
of clinicians, who consider they have more important things to do. It is,

of course, possible that the modes of analysis associated with scientific management persist in forums thus divorced from organisational arrangements based on associated precepts. This case study does not offer any information on this point. However, the next case study does and the two together can help us reach a more substantive judgement of the compatability of medical and managerial influences on the nature of health authorities and the relative influence of the two.

The Allocation of Beds for Geriatrics in a Teaching DGH[11]

This case study (to which we referred in Chapter 3) concerns a provincial DGH in the process of massive redevelopment. The particular focus was the allocation of beds in Phase III which, at the time of the study, was expected to be commissioned in three years' time. Like all studies of decision-making, this case is complicated by the multiplicity of interconnected aspects, for example, in this case by the teaching needs of the various specialties. The assumptions on which the decisions were made also changed dramatically midway through the case study. At the start of the study, participants were optimistic about future invest-ment and claims unmet in the development nearing completion could be met in Phase IV, which would materialise in the foreseeable future. In the middle of the study period these assumptions were radically challenged. Economic problems, a loan from the International Mone-tary Fund and a deflationary budget resulted in 'cuts' in the capital budget. Given these complications, we looked at the decision-making process from the point of view of geriatrics, around which the major controversy raged. We also narrowed the focus to the issues as seen by one DMT, though there was (and is) considerable interdependency with services administered by another DMT in the same city.

The District Medical Committee, as in the previous study, was virtually redundant and the dialogues between the DMT and the hospital consultants was conducted through the medium of the Medical Execu-tive Committee. However, the balance between it and the divisions was somewhat different. The latter were the effective decision-making agencies and the committee tended to act as post-box between them and the DMT. In the district there were active divisions of psychiatry, medicine, surgery, paediatrics, radiology, pathology and anaesthetics. The one consultant in geriatrics (plus another locum) was a member of the division of medicine. As we shall see below, this combination created no problems when both General Medicine and Geriatrics seemed assured of development but changed when there was a conflict of interests. At that point, the division represented the interests of the general physicians rather than the geriatrician.

It will be recalled that geriatrics was one of the beneficiaries of the central policy on priorities in the NHS. One aspect was incorporation of geriatric facilities into the new DGHs and specific targets were set. The principle was also to apply to the prestigious teaching hospitals, traditionally the great centres of medical research and training in the high-technology specialties. This followed logically from their growing responsibilities for a general district service. Furthermore, it was seen as important that doctors in training should also learn about the commoner problems in medicine.

Narrative. Phase II of the development (about 200 hospital beds) had been custom-built for geriatrics but had been occupied, on a temporary basis, by patients of the general physicians. Their accommodation had been demolished to allow the building of Phase III of the project to proceed. The provisional bed allocation for Phase III included 90 for geriatric assessment in its complement of 500 plus. The remainder were allocated largely to the surgical specialties, with 125 beds for maternity cases. Phase IV was intended for general medicine which would permit the temporary occupation of geriatric facilities to end.

The DMT began the process of getting agreement on the final alloca-tion of beds in Phase III by proposing three options, *none* of which made any provision for geriatric assessment. The rationale was the development of geriatric facilities in the other district which reduced the number of such beds needed to 60; the opening of an annexe near other acute facilities within the same district before Phase III was com-missioned and the opportunity to achieve another widely desired objec-tive – the centralisation of maternity services in the district. The increase in the number of maternity beds was also thought to be more consistent with the surgical emphasis of this particular part of the development.

The DMTs proposals were sent to the Medical Executive Committee who passed them on to its constituent divisions with support for a particular option. The divisions of surgery, radiology and paediatrics, while some had comments on the issues affecting their own specialty, did not demur from the recommendation of the executive committee: another, anaesthetics, without such a direct interest, merely 'received' and 'noted' the report. The reservations came from divisions of medicine (whose responsibilities encompassed geriatrics), psychiatry and the nursing division of geriatrics. The latter objected to the associ-ated idea of upgrading wards in a block some distance from the main facilities and said that the gains in staffing resulting from an earlier transfer to a central block would be lost. The division of medicine asked for the reinstatement of the 60 geriatric assessment beds in Phase III.

When the Medical Executive Committee came to consider these views they also had further comments from the district administrator. He felt that the development of the geriatric service, together with the commitment to give the upgrading of old, separate accommodation on the DGH site top priority, gave 'rise to the risk of disturbing the balance of service to all other specialties'. He wished to avoid the acute services 'becoming the deprived specialties of the future', and pointed to the longer waiting lists for admission than for the geriatric service. Furthermore, it was important to get maternity services out of an isolated unit.

The outcome of these exchanges of view (the CHC had also expressed opposition to the exclusion of geriatric assessment beds from Phase III) was a compromise proposal: there were to be 30 geriatric assessment beds. The paper outlining the final recommendation (to the AHA(T)) contained comments very relevant to our interest in the nature of the local process. It talked of 'constraints on the DMT from all levels, which could have rapidly resulted in a polyglot situation defying decision', and said that the recommendation 'represented a considered and calculated decision for the bed allocations in Phase III, following comprehensive discussions with all interested parties'. The proposals were approved by the AHA(T) and passed on to the RHA for approval.

RHA approval was *not* forthcoming – a decision that received direct backing from the DHSS itself. Although the RHA accepted the need for centralisation of obstetric services (a proposal in line with DHSS policy), particularly because of the high neonatal mortality rates, it rejected the method of achieving it, especially the repeated relegation of geriatrics from accommodation planned for its use to that abandoned by other specialties. They argued that Phase III had to be considerably more than a temporary solution because an early start on Phase IV was unrealistic in the current economic climate. Furthermore, an HAS team report towards the end of the previous year had been extremely critical of the district's geriatric services. It had rejected the DMT's proposal to place the 90 geriatric beds in the accommodation in the old block away from the main facilities. The RHA insisted on at least 60 geriatric beds being provided in Phase III, if the difference of 30 could be located in accommodation elsewhere with convenient access to diagnostic and therapeutic facilities. The DMT's aim of centralising other services from peripheral hospitals (like maternity) could still be achieved if parts of the accommodation on the old site were retained and upgraded now that Phase IV was unlikely to happen (at least for a long time). This postponement also raised the question of the resiting of the General Medical Unit to 'honour the previous under-taking that Phase II would revert to geriatric rehabilitation at the earliest possible stage'.

The local negotiations clearly had to begin again. They were to be centred around both the bed allocation for Phase III and a wing of the hospital (centrally sited) now to be retained (not the one in which it had been proposed to rehouse the geriatric assessment beds). A number of bids for a share of the central accommodation preceded the start of the new process in which the DMT and Medical Executive Committee worked together very closely. Both considered a discussion document simultaneously, suggesting the return of Phase II to geriatrics and 60 assessment beds in Phase III. The latter involved shifting the provision for two specialties to the centrally sited old block.

The divisions were again invited to comment. Most accepted the new proposals though not without reservations. The division of surgery, for example, objected to the reductions in beds proposed for gynaecology. The major objections now came from the division of medicine which put in a claim for general medical beds in Phase III since the next phase was now unlikely to proceed until the end of the century. The physicians pushed their objections to losing their facilities in Phase II without some better alternative hard and called a special meeting. The outcome of this pressure was an agreement by the Medical Executive Committee that the general medical unit would continue to be housed in Phase II and that the revised proposals for Phase III be accepted, with some small adjustments in the allocation of beds to the surgical specialties.

The DHSS had made its position clear in the middle of these exchanges. It had endorsed the recommendations of the HAS team report and pointed out that even if 90 beds in Phase III were allocated to geriatrics, this could mean that only 18 per cent of the geriatric beds in the district were located centrally on the DGH site, compared with the interim target of 30 per cent. The argument that the geriatric beds in (upgraded) old accommodation and in the new purpose-built devel-opment elsewhere should be classified as being located on the DGH/ teaching site was rejected since the facilities would not have direct access to diagnostic and therapeutic departments. The proposal to convert an obstetric into a geriatric hospital when obstetric services were centralised was also unacceptable. When the district administrator wrote informing his area colleague of this local agreement he referred to pressure from the DHSS in spite of which they had decided that only 60 assessment beds were required for geriatrics. Nevertheless, he suggested that a further meeting with RHA and DHSS officials would be of benefit if the dispute about bed allocations were to continue. In fact, with some caveats, the proposals were accepted at that stage thus allowing the commissioning work to proceed.

The Case Study: Preliminary Comment. While the formal exchanges represent only one element in what was clearly a very intensive exercise, they are nevertheless sufficient to point to the kind of impact doctors had on these decisions and the role of the Cogwheel machinery. The picture is, in fact, very clear. The role of the Medical Executive Committee was primarily a political one. The important thing was to get agreement between parties concerned. The DMT played a similar role, spurred on by the need for definitive decisions as quickly as possible to allow the commissioning process to proceed smoothly.

The Impact of Medical Staff on the Nature of Local Health Systems

The earlier discussion pointed to intended harmonies between the formal management arrangements for the NHS and the structure for medical participation. Both were informed by a particular view on the appropriate distribution of authority (hierarchy), how decisions should be made (rational analysis) and the values (efficiency etc.) to which greater weight needed to be given. If the harmonies were found to exist in practice, it would suggest that the nature of health authorities and their sub-units (and local policy outcomes) could be best understood by adopting a managerialist framework.

The material in this and the previous chapter, however, does not support such a contention. If it had, it could then have been argued that the NHS was unique. In few organisations would it be claimed that the precepts associated with scientific management, as manifested in formal arrangements, were the overwhelming influence on what actually happened. The material suggests rather the reverse — the difference between practice and theory is such that we can conclude that in these cases other influences were much more important.

It is, of course, possible that the differences were not due to the incompatibilities of the management and medical ways of doing things, values etc., but inadequate design of arrangements for participation, or inappropriate implementation. Goldsmith and Mason have suggested that one condition of effectiveness is divisions of a viable size that contain a workable grouping of specialists.[12] In the first case study, this condition was not met. Both districts were small, divisions had consequently to be all-embracing and the allocation of specialties was consequently seen as arbitrary. For example, in the district where obstetrics was allocated to the surgical and paediatrics to the medical division, any dialogues between the two must have gone against the grain of the Cogwheel structure. In small districts, divisions have to be constituted that are representative of specialty interests but are too small to be viable, or are large enough to be viable but are unrepresentative of specialty interests.

Even in larger districts, as in the second case study, the marriages of specialties can cause problems. The interests of geriatrics and general physicians diverged as the disagreement about the allocation of beds in Phase III of the DGH development deepened and champions of the former emerged from other parts of the system. The divisional structure was unable to cope with this conflict and the Medical Executive Committee had to negotiate a compromise.

Goldsmith and Mason further argue that another condition of effectiveness is that potential participants, especially consultants, have to believe they have something to gain from the divisional arrangement. They argue, perhaps tautologically, that 'to the extent that divisions can evade unpopular action or difficult decisions, or that individuals withhold their co-operation, the system cannot work effectively'. Or to put it another way, if medical practitioners resist co-option into the management structure, there is very little anybody can do about it. In the first case study doctors were prepared to be co-opted only on their own terms and in a forum constructed and controlled by themselves. When these conditions were not met (e.g. in district medical committees), the machinery became redundant.

A second factor in the failure of divisions and District Medical Committees also points to a certain degree of incompatibility between medical and management models of behaviour. The structure in the first case study appears to have been seen by medical practitioners as alien and imposed and either unrepresentative or outside the control of the constituent members. In both districts the consultants substituted in place of divisions less formal systems (clinical meetings and journal clubs) amenable to more direct control. These had a clear-cut clinical rationale, were voluntary and self-instituted and were not perceived as a waste of time.

A similar set of factors maintained the Medical Executive and prevented the development of the District Medical Committee. Executive or advisory committees of hospital doctors, especially consultants, have existed for a long time. The more optional nature of Medical Executive Committees and the freedom to change their constitution at will, seems to increase the sense of involvement with it. The authors of the Grey Book, aware that they might create too many medical committees, had suggested that it be removed from the administrative hierarchy and given the status of an optional sub-committee of the District Medical Committee. However, consultants in the first case study maintained the importance and status of the Medical Executive Committee, with only a token representation of other groups. It was the only body by whose decision they felt bound. In the second case study, the negotiations with doctors were also channelled only through the Medical Executive Committee, though in that case the divisions were much stronger.

The differences in the DGH case study between the functions and process assumed in the formal model and reality are particularly interesting. Goldsmith and Mason envisage the most successful medical management structures emerging in this kind of situation since problems of size of division and internal coherence are reduced. Defects in design or implementation are thus unconvincing explanations of discrepancies. Their existence reinforces our earlier suggestions of elements of incompatibility between the management and medical systems and the pre-eminence of the latter.

There is a superficial similarity between the eventual outcome (geriatric assessment beds were to be provided in Phase III) and the logic of a central policy that had received general assent throughout the service. It was, however, largely explained by the intervention of outside agencies rather than managerialism. Left to itself, the local political market would have perhaps produced 30 beds and that would not have owed much to conviction. The important determinants were power of the different provider groups who used the policies, norms of provision, priorities and targets as the 'chips' in the game. They presented the bits that fitted a case based on perceptions of interest and ideology of the group concerned: they did not have much persuasive power in their own right. The outcome was the product of bargaining between groups (including the centre) and is a fair measure of the power of each of the participants.

This description of how decisions involving medical staff were reached is at odds with the notions of structure and process on which the management arrangements for the service are based. It suggests a system that has much in common with the incrementalist theories of Lindblom,[13] to which we return in the final chapter. For example, the analysis did not, as far as we could discern, separate out value goals and empirical analysis. The two were intertwined rather than the 'clarification of values of objectives' prior to the consideration of alternative courses of action. The latter process, according to Lindblom, is characteristic of rational modes of decision-making, while the former describes the incrementalist approach. Another similarity is the criterion used to assess the rightness of the policy. The incrementalist test is agreement between interested parties rather than the choice of the option most likely to realise previously agreed ends. This describes well the search for agreement among the interested parties about the allocation of beds in Phase III.

An immediate objection to this line of argument, however, is the representativeness of our case studies. How do we know other health authorities work in the same way? In short, we do not know, but the analysis here offers a hypothesis against which to test experience in other health authorities. Comments made by Perrin in his report to the Royal Commission, however, suggests that the experiences described here are not unique:

> Clinicians may be so formidable as to dominate decisions about resource use . . . the exercise of clinical autonomy ought not be allowed to extend to a veto on reallocation of beds to cope with changes in need. We came across a flagrant example of such a veto . . . [14]

Medical dominance of the local decision-making process is, of course, hardly a revelation, especially to those who work in the NHS. Our argument, however, is slightly different. It is that the local health authorities will be influenced by *different* ideas about ways of working (structure, process) and which values should be given the highest priority. The ideas about structure, process and values that inform the formal management arrangements are only one set of influences, and others, such as the different ideology and interests of clinicians, are more important. These differences produce a political situation in which differential power is important. The actual role of mechanisms established to promote rational-man type analyses are thus converted into forums for negotiation, bargaining, compromise and the promotion of consensus. This is true both of the management teams in the previous chapter and the Medical Executive Committee in this. Perrin suggests that this is also true of health authorities which 'tend to have to resolve disputes rather than apply its time considering . . . what would be in the best interests of health care in the area'.[15]

In the case of doctors the evidence here suggests that the Cogwheel reports and the 1974 reorganisation of the health service did not radically alter the pattern of involvement in management. The pattern remained one of informal rather than formal co-option. In other words, the medical profession, and more especially the acute hospital specialists, maintained effective power without concomitant responsibility. Arguments about the declining power of the medical profession because of the rising power of administrators or unionised unskilled labour are as premature as arguments about the increasing managerial penetration and resulting unionisation of the medical profession.

Where then does this leave our argument? We have suggested that the use health authorities (or any other agency that replaces them) make of the action space available to them will be determined by what we have called the nature of local systems. The material in this chapter has suggested that one important influence is the different views and interests of the groups that compose it and that the resolution of differences, particularly when the medical profession is concerned, is via a political rather than a scientific-type managerial process. It also suggests, at least as far as issues that have implications for them are concerned, that the medical view provides the ideological framework in which others work. The medical view of what the local service is all about prevails and is accepted by others. Furthermore, that medical view has not been seduced by the advent of scientific management structures into accepting the primacy of its associated values; the formal management arrangements provide the forums and language for what remains an essentially political process. An understanding of the health authorities (and the NHS) therefore requires a thorough examination of the different facets of the political process at work to see, for example, if the local systems are as elitist in nature as our argument has suggested.

Notes

1. This chapter is a revised version of a paper read at the annual meeting of the Medical Sociology Group of the British Sociological Association by

A. Alaszewski, D. Vulliamy, T. Matus and T. James, 'Doctors and Management: Co-opted or Co-opting', York, 22-24 September 1978.

2. Ministry of Health, *First Report of the Joint Working Party on the Organisation of Medical Work in Hospitals*, Chairman, Sir G. Godber (HMSO, London, 1967). Specific references in this section are (in sequence) to paras. 29, 58, 62, 69, 11 and 71.

3. DHSS, *Second Report of the Joint Working Party on the Organisation of Medical Work in Hospitals* (HMSO, London, 1972). Specific references in this section are (in sequence) to p. 39, paras. 7.17-7.19, 4.5, 4.6, 4.9, 4.1, 4.10, 5.6, 5.4 and 5.6.

4. DHSS, *Management Arrangements for the Reorganised National Health Service* (HMSO, London, 1972), para. 2.42.

5. Ibid., para. 2.55.

6. Ministry of Health, *Report of the Committee on Senior Nursing Staff Structure*, Chairman, B. Salmon (HMSO, London, 1966; National Board for Prices and Incomes, *The Pay and Conditions of Services of Ancillary Workers in the National Health Service*, Report No. 166, Cmnd. 4644 (HMSO, London, 1971).

7. P. Selznick, *TVA and the Grass Roots* (University of California Press, Berkeley, 1953), p. 13.

8. A. Flanders, *Management and the Unions* (Faber & Faber, London, 1970), p. 172.

9. The material was collected by M. Lee and T. Matus for a project conducted by the Institute for Health Studies, University of Hull, financed by the Nuffield Provincial Hospitals Trust.

10. See for example, O. Goldsmith and A. Mason, *Information for Action* (Joint Working Party on the Organisation of Medical Work in Hospitals, DHSS, 1974).

11. The material was collected by T. James and R. Chandler for a project conducted by the Institute for Health Studies, University of Hull, financed by the Social Science Research Council.

12. Goldsmith and Mason, *Information for Action*, pp. 2-5.

13. C.E. Lindblom, 'The Science of "Muddling Through" ', *Public Administration Review*, vol. 19 (Spring 1959), pp. 79-88.

14. Royal Commission on the National Health Service, 'Management of Financial Resources in the National Health Service', *Research Paper*, No. 2 (HMSO, London, 1978), para. B7.6.

15. Ibid., para. B8.24.

7 THE NHS: THE WAY FORWARD

We began this book by saying that change strategies had been misconceived, because they ignored the local dimension in the NHS. Without a more complete model of how the service works, change strategies will remain defective. In this final chapter we sketch out some of the theoretical implications of our approach and the kind of change strategy that flows from it.

The Need for a Theory

It is one thing to demonstrate the inadequacy of a theory of the NHS based on managerial models of behaviour. It is quite another to offer a comprehensive alternative, particularly when there is no one accepted theory of organisation. Even where there is a wealth of empirical material on the internal dynamics of an organisation, there are a number of competing perspectives (e.g. human relations, closed or open systems, contingency etc.) and there is no generally acceptable synthesis in sight. In an organisation such as the NHS, with unique features and its internal dynamics scarcely explored, a comprehensive theory is even further away.

Nevertheless, it is important that a start be made, though there are sceptics within the service who would not accord such an activity any priority at all. For some, the words 'theory' and 'academic' have a perjorative flavour. Some are particularly suspicious of new insights emanating from the social sciences. They do not fit their traditional orientation to the biological sciences and often these theories challenge the dominant position of the professional in the division of labour and their control of the practitioner-patient relationship. A common reaction is to dismiss these notions and argue for the 'good old days'.[1] Yet it is no good hankering after the 'golden age' of the voluntary hospital, the group secretary and the matron. The simpler informal relationships cannot be revived in what is now a completely different situation. Practitioners cannot reject all contributions from the social sciences, which are especially relevant to the new institutions of social welfare and the impact of large organisations. They must learn to choose between the good, useful and bad theories.

The case for disregarding the scepticism of the practical man is overwhelming. The material in the book has underlined how this sentiment can be an insurmountable obstacle to successful change. The 1974 reorganisation is but one testimony to the futility of basing change strategies on partial or erroneous theories of how the NHS and its constituent parts actually work. The adoption of such arrangements as corporate management, for example, can only be explained by reference to a theory in which managers have a much more positive role than we have described. The secondary, supportive, consensus-building role of teams readily discernible in our material, also means that the managers' definitions of important problems for attention should be cautiously received. Managers who assume that their own preoccupations are shared by other participants in their unit, sector or district because they are *the* managers, are likely to miscue and thus evoke the wrong response. Managers in the NHS are not the dominant force that they seem to be in the allegedly non-theoretical, commonly accepted assumptions of the everyday world. If they believe this, it is because they are mistakenly applying to the NHS models of management developed in the private sector.

There are fairly obvious examples of how concepts based on non-medical theories can help us understand some aspect of NHS development, or the relationships within and between health authorities. One example of 'useful' theory is the link between the growth of trade union activity and changes in management structure and the suggestion that managers can and do find unions useful in their search for more control.[2] This view of labour relations explains a lot of the actions of managers and increasing unionisation within the NHS without having to resort to the approach that focuses *exclusively* on the personalities involved, the local situation and the calibre of managers. Again, a modest knowledge of economics would have been sufficient to have warned practitioners, a decade before, of the likely 'plateau' in public expenditure in the 1970s. It would also eliminate much of the surprise of many at 'windfalls' or short-term cutbacks. A little knowledge of economic concepts, which increases the appreciation of likely trends in public expenditure, makes a *practical* contribution to the management of resources in the NHS by reducing uncertainty.

These homely examples on the value of wider perspectives, however, only serve to underline the absence of a general framework which explains crucial developments. We have referred to the way additional resources were used in English hospitals between 1970 and 1977. Managerial 'commonsense' might have had us believe that the increases would have been used to treat more patients. Another example is the experience of the services for the mentally ill. How can we explain the failure of health agencies to give them a higher priority when it was clear that this was one of the growing problem areas of the NHS? Similarly, there is as yet no convicing explanation for the different pattern of industrial relations and actions in various parts of the country.

We hasten to add that we have no comprehensive theory of the NHS to offer. What we have tried to do is point to some starting points for such an enterprise. These include the considerable power of the local agency; the consequent need to draw on studies with a 'local perspective', as well as a centralist one; the significance of the 'political system' of health agencies in decision-making; the consequent need to draw on concepts of power, interest and values to explain local processes and outcomes; the need to explain variations between (and indeed within) health agencies in positive terms and not resort to negative features such as 'breakdowns in communication', 'misunderstandings' or inadequate mechanisms of control; and the non-directive character of management in the NHS.

We now turn to two of these issues, the power of the medical profession and the likely nature of the management process in health agencies. The objectives are to relate our material to discussion of wider issues and indicate the kind of concepts that might be found useful in studies of health agencies. The approach is eclectic, drawing on different perspectives. Like Hunter[3] (who has also studied the decision-making in health agencies), we quote Rein in justification: 'Major paradigms contain stories which describe intrinsically good ways of looking at reality . . . These are persuasive whether or not we accept the whole paradigm of thought from which they come.'[4] Since there is no *one* theory of organisation, the eclectic approach is not only inevitable but has the blessing of utility for students of health agencies.

The Medical Profession and Concepts of Power

The assertion that the medical profession is powerful, locally as well as nationally, naturally comes as no surprise to NHS personnel, sociologists, civil servants or politicians. Nevertheless, it is worth noting in passing that the Royal Commission was made very much aware of doctors' fears that their 'status' was declining. Apparently, clinicians feel threatened by the growth of paramedical groups and their claims to areas of competence and autonomy, as well as by managers.[5]

It is presumably these feelings that have contributed to problems

between pathologists and laboratory scientists.[6] The identification of
the latter as budget-holders for laboratories with the implication of
overall managerial responsibility, is being resisted by pathologists who
have now developed an enthusiasm for courses in management. In
some areas of the country the difficulties between the two groups have
become acute, with threats of industrial action by the scientists. There
are other groups with whom relationships are difficult (not necessarily
at individual level) even if the problems are not so obvious. The
response of the medical profession is to concede the necessity for interdisciplinary working but under the leadership of a clinician.

In spite of the fear of the profession, the research material has
indicated a continuing medical hegemony in important decisions
within the NHS. This observation, however, does not take our analysis
of the power of the doctors any further. We need to know how far and
how often the clinical 'writ' runs in the local management of the service
and its nature. Does it, for example, really extend as far as the management of the laundry? And what about the content of plans? The
answers to these and many other questions require the student of the
health service to explore the notion of power beyond the simple definition offered earlier in the book:

> The capacity of an individual, or a group of individuals, to modify
> the conduct of other individuals or groups in the manner which he
> desires and to prevent his own being modified in the manner he does
> not.[7]

This definition is, nevertheless, useful as a starting point because it
draws attention to the idea of power as a relationship between individuals or groups. Power is also seen to have a positive dimension (control
exercised by one group over another) and a negative one (the autonomy
or independence of one group from another). Medical practitioners
possess the second type of power in their freedom from managerial
control and clinical autonomy. In contrast, ancillary workers have never
had this autonomy and there seems to have been a considerable erosion
of the autonomy of ward sisters following the Salmon Report. There is,
however, little evidence of a similar trend in medicine.

The use of this notion of power in studies of groups within health
authorities does not tell us much about the factors that influence and
determine its use. Lukes has described the definitions of power that
focus only on behaviour as one-dimensional. He argues that this view
focuses on '*behaviour* in the making of *decisions* on *issues* over which

there is an observable *conflict* of (subjective) *interests*, seen as express policy preferences, revealed by political participation'.[8] In this one-dimensional framework the important factors are:

  (i)   the identity of the groups;

 (ii)   the issues over which they are in conflict;

(iii)   the rules of the game; and

(iv)   the resources that the different groups bring to bear in this game.

    The observable conflicts, and the light these throw on the use of power, are, however, probably only the tip of the iceberg. A more important use of power is control over the issues at stake and the rules of the game. If a group can maintain control of the agenda and prevent issues antipathetic to their interests reaching it, conflict is prevented and effective control maintained.

    Lukes defines this view as the two-dimensional approach to power. Its emphasis is also on non-decisions, which are defined as follows:

> a decision that results in suppression or thwarting of a latent or manifest challenge to the values or interests of the decision-maker . . . a means by which demands for change in the existing allocation of benefits and privileges in the community can be suffocated before they are even voiced; or kept covert or killed before they gain access to the relevant decision-making arena — or, failing all these things, maimed or destroyed in the decision-making stage of the policy process.[9]

    In the NHS, the agenda, especially at local level, has been controlled by the medical profession. Thus, local politics are medical politics. The upper reaches of the NHS may be more open to new policy initiatives, but these are rapidly filtered. By the time they reach the local agency, they have been readjusted to fit into the local political agenda. This can be seen most clearly in the planning system which was an attempt, by the centre, to change the way in which the local political agenda was formed. The guidance made it clear, for example, that consideration should be extended to existing commitments as possible sources of monies for needed developments. The centre also tried to use the planning system to put the case for the cinderella services firmly on the local agendas. Our description of these efforts suggests that they can hardly be said to have been a resounding success. The proper designation is really 'failed', particularly since public expenditure plans for 1980/1 envisage an absolute decline in spending by Social Service Departments. They are responsible for developing community services which are disproportionately used by cinderella groups, and the cut-back in resources indicates an abandonment of the effective priority for them. It is another recognition of the centre's inability to have an effective influence on the local agenda.

It is, of course, possible to point to the great numbers of people other than clinicians now involved in the planning process. The planning system, and other features of the 1974 arrangements for the NHS, were intended to draw groups into the management system. Participation was the keyword, and the frequent complaints about over-consultation suggest that it has been put into effect. Certainly there are opportunities for participation for groups not previously involved in planning service development. How can this development be reconciled with our conclusion of continuing medical hegemony within local systems, largely insulated from pressure from the centre and the local environment? Or put more directly, why don't administrators, for example, have more power? Why don't they have more influence on the agenda? In concrete terms, why do the consensus teams react rather than initiate?

The sociologists' conceptualisation of power again offers some explanations. The two- rather than one-dimensional model is an improvement since it directs attention to non-decision, the process by which issues are excluded from the agenda. However, it still focuses on conflict and behaviour. As Lukes points out, this ignores 'the crucial point that the most effective and insidious use of power is to prevent such conflict from arising in the first place'.[10] The most effective use of power is to control the production of ideas, and ensure that only a version of reality that favours the interests of a specific group exists.

> Is it not the supreme and most insidious exercise of power to prevent people, to whatever degree, from having grievances by shaping their perceptions, cognitions and preferences in such a way that they accept their role in the existing order of things, either because they can see or imagine no alternative to it, or because they see it as natural and unchangeable or because they value it as divinely ordained and beneficial?[11]

This is undoubtedly the primary source of medical power. The so-called medical model of disease defines the purpose of health service personnel: the emphasis is on putting right clinically defined ill health, and no other group has offered a clear alternative prospectus. The first part of this observation is a commonplace, agreed by authors as widely divergent as Culyer, Klein, Freidson and Illich.

The lack of an articulated alternative prospectus is, however, not so generally recognised. The Unit for the Study of Health Policy, in its examination of the role of the mass media, points out that health has become unequivocally equated with the consumption of health services.

> The pinnacle of achievement in health has come to be equated with the spectacle of men and women becoming overstressed and under-exercised, indulging in excessive consumption of food, cigarettes and alcohol for a number of years, before being rushed to an intensive care unit and submerged in expensive medical technology only when acute symptoms have prevented them from indulging in further consumption.[12]

The unit argues for a broader agenda including:
   (i)   promoting health in a positive sense;
  (ii)   primary prevention;
 (iii)   assistance with and facilitation of natural processes;
 (iv)   managing existing health problems;
  (v)   spreading an understanding of health and health care; and
 (vi)   providing personal support in relation to health problems.[13]
Only the fourth item is on the current agenda of local health agencies.

The insulation of health agencies from local environmental and central influences means that an alternative view of their role must obtain the backing of participants in the local political system. One view (essentially Marxist) is that this would only happen when the group concerned saw that its own interest, and that of the class of society with which it identified, coincided with the alternative view. Crudely, NHS personnel can be divided into three such groups — doctors, managers and other workers, with members of authorities and paramedics in a somewhat ambiguous position. This view would identify the medical profession with the owners of capital, the bulk of the NHS with the working class (the position of paramedical workers would be similar to that of the middle class and share similar tensions), and the managers with the state. If this type of association was accepted, then groups inside the NHS would be concerned not only with their immediate self-interest, i.e. control over the conditions and content of work, but would, at the same time, act as agents for the equivalent group outside the NHS. Navarro has attempted to establish this type of relationship.[14]

At the national level, it is possible to detect the development of alternative ideologies in, for example, the policies of central government. They have been concerned with the redistribution of resources from acute, high-technology medicine to the cinderella services and with ever-increasing emphasis on prevention and health education. These concerns indicate a different prospectus for health services. To date, local managers have not been persuaded of the validity of this alternative. Similarly, signs of a broader agenda, particularly in the emphasis on prevention of ill health, in some union evidence to the Royal Commission[15] contrasts with the limited, conservative and defensive reactions of local representatives.

Services for the mentally handicapped provide a good example of the reaction of different interest groups and the problems for the cinderellas in a medically orientated NHS. The leadership of the medical profession apparently does not see mental handicap as a medical responsibility and would probably prefer to see it transferred from the NHS to local authority Social Services Departments. The Central Health Services Council reports on the functions of the DGH, locates assessment services there, places a small number in traditional mental handicap hospitals and the majority in community care.[16] As there are only about 100 consultant psychiatrists in mental subnormality, the impact of this specialism on the local medical political system tends to be marginal. The government's proposals have been set out in a White Paper, *Better Services for the Mentally Handicapped*,[17] and in a document on priorities. There is also the report of a working party (Jay) on the subject.[18] To some extent all three follow the thinking of medical profession. The bulk of services should be provided by Social Services Departments, but until they develop real alternatives there should be a shift of resources to the mental handicap sector in the NHS and the traditional large hospital should be broken up. The union attitude has been reactive, defensive and concerned with the impact on jobs. Given this constellation of local forces, it is not surprising that there is little evidence that managers accept either the high priority or the need for smaller community orientated facilities.

We are, however, in uncharted territory because power and the concept of interest (and values — which we have not discussed) has not been given a more prominent place in analyses of health agencies.We are consequently unsure of the precise perceptions of interest and value held by groups and thus the (in)validity of resorting to frameworks based on general views of society. This also applies to the use of power in the field and the mechanisms for its use, with the result that one potentially potent explanation for change (or the lack of it) in a particular setting has been ignored. Power is not a constant commodity and changes in its configuration might explain changes in local behaviour.

The preceding all too brief allusions to concepts of power in the context of health agencies has, we hope, indicated their utility to the student of the NHS. Rather than being seen as distasteful features of life that should not apply to the caring services (except perhaps when one's own position is in question), the notions of power, interest and values must be brought firmly and openly into the spotlight of enquiry. Until they are, we shall continue to misunderstand a key factor in the nature of local health agencies in the NHS.

The Nature of the Management Process in Health Agencies

The nature of management in a health agency will reflect – perhaps be dependent – on the local configurations of power, perceptions of interest and values of its constituent groups. An appreciation of the role of managers and the management process will therefore be enhanced by the use of a political framework for analysis. In saying this we must be careful not to throw the baby out with the bathwater. The management arrangements remain a factor in local behaviour, and the concepts developed to describe them will therefore have to remain within the remit of the analyst. The view taken here is that it will be profitable (on the basis of our field material) to relegate them to a minor role in studies of health agencies, and replace them with concepts originating in studies of administrative politics. It will be noted, too, that we still do not advocate the adoption of a particular set of ideas. We persist in our eclectic approach, using concepts that seem of value in a particular context.

The idea that political relations between groups are a more important factor in behaviour than those prescribed in the management arrangements is, of course, hardly new. It is a familiar theme in much of the literature on organisations. While it still remains unfamiliar in studies of health authorities, the need to adopt such a perspective has been recognised by some recent authors. Dimmock and Barnard have argued for the recognition of 'sectional interests' as a necessary ingredient of 'an accurate description of inter-group relations within the service or relationships with the environment'.[19] Hunter, in a study of decisions on the use of development funds in two Scottish health boards, also makes use of concepts drawn from studies of administrative politics.[20]

The use of a political framework does not imply that health authorities are in a perpetual state of internal conflict. Studies of RHA decisions on the allocation of monies to AHAs in the late 1970s would hardly substantiate such a view. There was disquiet, debate and deputations over the speed with which allocations should be moved towards their RAWP targets and special compensation ended for additional revenue costs arising out of capital developments. The strong association between the authorities' views of the wisdom of the formula for allocations (favourable/unfavourable) and its effect on them (higher/standstill budgets) indicates how strong the perception of interest was in these exchanges. Yet, in spite of the centrality of the final decisions to the fortune of health authorities, the debate never got out of hand.[21]

The absence of overt conflict in our material (though not, of course, in the case of Lambeth, Southwark and Lewisham AHA(T)) does not, however, invalidate the use of a political perspective to explain behaviour. It rather directs attention to the local operating procedures and understandings about process and priorities, and in turn to their origins. Strauss *et al.* have suggested the notion of 'negotiated order' as a model for understanding the emergence of 'shared agreements, the binding contracts – which constitute the grounds for our expectable, non-surprising, taken-for-granted, even ruled orderliness', which all change over time.[22] This was based on work on two psychiatric hospitals in the USA some years ago, but Hunter has more recently argued that the politics of decision-making are also about the operation of routines and standard operating procedures.[23] These procedures have a *political* significance, and it is their legitimacy that is an important factor in avoiding overt conflict.

The complexity of issues facing health authorities is another factor that directs attention to political activities rather than the 'cognitive deficiencies' of the participants.[24] There are different objectives to which different groups will give different priorities; there is no criterion that enables an unchallengeable decision to be made on, for example, the relative merits of additional investment in the neurological or geriatric service: the uncertainties (e.g. in likely advances in medical technology) preclude precise evaluations of likely opportunities, costs or outcomes of particular developments. It is not surprising that Hunter drew attention to the 'puzzlement factor' in decision on the deployment of development funds by the two Scottish health boards. Where there is such complexity and puzzlement, the rational-man explanation for local behaviour is unlikely to be convincing. The decisions are likely to reflect the bargains struck, or understandings between groups, and do the minimum violence to the status quo.

This leads naturally on to the now popular theory of incrementalism as a useful framework for studies of health authorities. The
theory starts from the generally accepted premiss that rational decision-
making is impossible. People are unable to classify and rank values or
objectives, identify and evaluate alternative ways of realising them, and
be sufficiently confident of their effect to choose the 'right' one.
Unlike the rational decision-making enthusiasts, who, nevertheless,
proceed to use this unattainable model as a guide to behaviour,
Lindbolm (his name is synonymous with incrementalism) makes a
virtue of 'muddling through'. The mixing of empirical analysis and
consideration of values and objectives, the restricted analysis and the
successive limited comparisons, which he argues characterise real life,
are seen to have considerable advantages, including building on policies
that have been proved in practice, and avoiding major errors.[25]

One feature of the incrementalist perspective that merits a special
mention is the notion of mutual adjustment. It is particularly relevant
to the earlier discussion about the ways groups affect each other in
the policy-making process. 'Mutual adjustment is more pervasive than
the explicit forms it takes in negotiation between groups: it persists
through the mutual impacts of groups upon each other even when they
are not in communication.'[26] Attention is also directed to the groups
that exist and their influence: these are the factors that explain outcomes.

There are legitimate criticisms of incrementalism. It is never clear
whether a particular policy is incremental or not. Does the creation of
Community Health Councils in 1974, for example, fall into the incremental category? Should incrementalism be commended when the rate
of scientific, economic and social change requires radical responses
from managers and policy-makers? Should the concept be applied
separately to process and outcomes? In spite of this deficiency, the
theory does evoke recognition from people within management and its
insights should be helpful in a study of health agencies, particularly
their political characteristics.

These descriptions of the *management* process in organisation certainly help us to appreciate the role of *managers* in the NHS. It explains
their preoccupation with process rather than policy-making, described
in Chapter 5. Managers 'manage' the mutual adjustment process to
ensure that it does not get out of hand. When an external party be-
comes involved such as the RHA, in the allocation of beds in a DGH
(Chapter 6), the managers arrange the accommodation between it and

the internal interests. The essentially reactive nature of management teams in the NHS described in the previous chapters also points to this kind of role for managers in the NHS.

This view of the managerial role (or more accurately an important component of it) directs attention to likely coping strategies to ensure a minimum of friction between local groups. The 'scapegoating' of higher authority is clearly one such strategy. The transfer *of odium* for the denial of an improvement is a useful way of maintaining local amity, even if those referring the issue upwards know it would be quite impossible to meet the request. The volume of complaints about the higher authority, the DHSS, the minister, the Treasury, is consistent with the view of local managers being primarily concerned with the maintenance of the equilibrium of the local system.

There are other strategies, one of which was present in the case study on the allocation of beds in the DGH. When a local decision had to be made between conflicting interests, the DMT identified with the interests of the strongest local group. In this case it was the acute consultants who gave a higher priority to the claims of obstetrics than to geriatrics, which had already been provisionally allocated space in the new development. Another strategy is ambiguity to avoid disputes and thus allow local groups to think that their interests have been protected. Some health authorities, for example, have approved strategic plans which require allocations well above the levels suggested in the indications of future revenue (planning assumptions). This tactic may, of course, constitute a bid for additional resources, but it also serves to leave unanswered questions of relative priority that could cause local dissension.

The concern of senior managers with the maintenance of an equilibrium between local groups is, of course, understandable. It is acknowledged to be a prime responsibility of management. The material on management teams in Chapter 5, the DGH case study in Chapter 6 and the nature of coping strategies that maximise local agreement, however, suggest something more. It suggests a preoccupation with this kind of activity, and it is this *preoccupation* that could be significant. We have taken it as a pointer to the nature of the managers' role, and thus the nature of the local system. If further work confirms this pattern of activity, it will strengthen our argument for the development of concepts based in administrative politics in studies of health agencies.

The suggestion that the role of NHS *managers* is best understood as a mediating one in an essentially political system does not limit the scope of the enterprising and forceful personality. Brief visits to health authorities are sufficient to indicate considerable differences between managers with some having a significant influence on local developments. The argument here – and it is only a hypothesis – suggests that this is more likely to be the case when the managers are closely identified with the most powerful groups, who in turn perceive their usefulness. In other words, managers, by dint of sorting out problems, facilitating development or offering efficient management services (including relevant data), build up a stock of support from which they can draw to influence the provider. It follows from this that managers who either do not offer efficient back-up services, or identify too closely with the interests of the cinderellas, will have less influence on the activities of acute consultants as a group. This will in turn limit the range of issues on which managers will have a significant influence. The essence of this view is the derivative nature of the influence of managers; it is not based on the centrality of their function to the activities of health agencies.

Comment

We have allowed ourselves to speculate on power and the role of managers beyond the boundaries of our empirical material. This was intentional because we wanted to demonstrate the insights that can come from enquiries of this type. The view that has dominated thinking about the NHS since its creation has neglected the political dimension and the deficiency needs to be remedied. Otherwise the picture of the management of the service will remain hopelessly partial. A fuller theory – in contradistinction to the sceptics mentioned at the beginning of the chapter – is thus the most effective way of offering practical help to those in the NHS.

Strategies for Change in the NHS

Where does this analysis leave the argument about change strategies in the NHS? It suggests that the latest reorganisation will, in itself, not facilitate ready responses to the changing circumstances in the 1980s and 1990s. The removal of the area tier of administration, the slimming down of management within districts, and government promises of less interference, will not change the basic nature of health agencies. They, or more accurately their providers, will continue to have a considerable impact on the pattern of development, and the local process of decision-making is still much more likely to resemble a political than a scientific management system. The ideology of the agency will continue to be provided by the local representatives of the medical profession, and particularly consultants in the acute specialties, with managers thrust into a brokerage rather than a directorate role. The other professionals will doubtless continue to strive for more personal autonomy and influence for their group and their successes and failures will be a factor in the precise texture of a local system at a particular point in time. The manual workers, if the present commitment to unions persists, will continue to have a capacity to hinder changes that are not in their interests. This will also be a variable commodity, thus injecting another local variable into the nature of the health agency.

There may be some who feel that this is a desirable state of affairs, and left to themselves health agencies will do as well without external interventions as with them. Certainly, our conclusions on the present state of affairs should encourage those who have criticised the allegedly growing power of managers over professional providers of service and have pressed for more decentralisation in government. While our material has undermined much of their analysis, evidence that their worst fears have proved unfounded should evoke a warm welcome. Nor should the rather different view of the realities in the NHS described here be taken as a barrier to their prescriptions for less management and central (or regional) interference. Since the centre's attempts to give a more positive lead have proved ineffective, it follows that the superstructures that originated in these developments are superfluous and could be removed. The changes proposed by the Conservative Government in 1979 fit in nicely with this line of argument.[27]

Problem Areas in Health Agencies

There are good reasons to think that the nature of many local agencies will, however, continue to inhibit ready and appropriate responses to some changes of circumstance. Two problem areas merit special attention. One stems from the distance of local providers from the national economic system. The total divorce of responsibility for raising cash and spending it, continues to fuel the fires of denigration so well described by Powell more than a decade ago. The system of central financing made it, in his view, ' a positive ethical duty [for providers] to besiege and bombard the government and force or shame them into providing more money, and then more again . . . '.[28] The Royal Commission's comment on the 'many . . . who gave evidence . . . that expenditure was nothing like enough'[29] suggests that little has changed.

Perhaps a more significant drawback, however, is insularity from local economic, social and political systems. Providers effectively control the amount of demand admitted into the system, the conditions to which they wish to accord priority, and investment in more diagnosis and therapy rather than increased throughput. Changes in the patterns of demand (and need) have, therefore, to be filtered through practitioners whose frames of reference might not be sympathetic to a ready response. The continued investment of a large slice of the annual increment in acute hospitals at a time when the numbers requiring services orientated to care rather than cure were increasing and those services needed funds to compensate for years of neglect is a case in point.

Insularity from the national economic system and changes in need cause problems for which some external compensation is necessary. Otherwise, responses will be more sluggish than they need be. It would be wrong to suggest an insensitivity to all kinds of changes in circumstances. There are some changes to which providers are very responsive, and those that affect medical practices in the acute field, in particular, fall into this category. In a review of advances in this field, the Royal Commission pointed to the

> impressive contribution which acute medicine has made in relieving
> illness and suffering . . . Diagnosis is continually being improved and
> refined by technological developments. Techniques such as tomography, ultrasound and radio-isotope scanning have been major
> advances. Analytical tools of great importance such as mass spectrometry, radio immunology and radioensymatic techniques have been
> added to the battery of 100 or more tests and investigations which a
> clinical laboratory in a district general hospital now provides.
> Advanced technology has contributed to the development of incubators for premature babies, renal transplantation, cardiac pacemakers
> and hip replacement. It is likely that bio-engineering will increasingly
> assist orthopaedics.[30]

This is an impressive list of changes that have been assimilated into medical practice in the NHS in a very short period of time. It is hardly indicative of a *general* unresponsiveness to change. The previous diagnosis of insularity refers to changes that do not correspond to the most powerful group's view of what medicine is all about. The (non-) response to challenges to the efficacy of some well-established medical interventions,[31] and arguments that alternative investments would be a more profitable way of improving health, are good illustrations of this unresponsive process at work. These notions are, of course, increasingly cogent in a situation of low growth rates and increasing costs of (usually) expensive developments. They also raise daunting ethical problems which again have not met with an eagerness to confront them.[32] These problems refer to the end products of health services. They also raise questions about the right balance of outputs and their relationships to the health status of the population (the real outcomes). These are the issues raised by changes in the circumstances of the NHS and where there is a need for a more rapid adjustment on the part of health authorities. This, in turn, requires an effective change strategy that will produce local conditions to facilitate appropriate and ready responses from local managers and providers.

Change strategies would also have to address themselves to another set of problems — those concerned with structure and process. We are not at this stage making many assumptions about the link between structure, process, outputs and outcomes, but want to raise the first two as problematical in their own right. The problems of structure and process are well documented in the voluminous literature on life in large-scale organisations. They include the problems of ensuring creativity, balancing the needs of specialisation with those of adequate co-ordination, information inadequacy and overload, and leadership.

One ill effect of the hierarchal structure in the NHS has been the centralised mentality of *some* officers. They expect decisions from above and are critical when their expectations are not met. There is some evidence that while promises of decentralisation are welcome in principle, they may be less welcome in practice.[33] When this is the case, a necessary condition of creativity is missing. The dynamic conservatism of staff in large organisations[34] can aso be expected to reinforce the factors that promote insularity from situational changes in health authorities.

The Essential Ingredients of a Change Strategy for the NHS

What kind of a strategy would effect the necessary changes in these problem areas of the NHS? We have already suggested that the current organisational changes will not be sufficient since they do little to compensate for the problems arising from the insularity of health agencies from certain aspects of their environment. Indeed, a policy of decentralisation unaccompanied by an ingredient that would either compensate for this factor or somehow remove it, could conceivably make the position worse in some places. The history of the NHS, however, warns us against taking professions by the centre of non-interference too seriously. Such promises have been made before and these have not

stood the test of time. Within weeks of taking office the present government, having put considerable emphasis on this aspect of their policy
for the NHS, nevertheless interfered with 'local' decisions about small
hospitals and the provision of office accommodation.[35] Whether or not
their resolve holds firm in the long run, the problem of the missing
ingredients in their strategy will remain.

The ground-rules for a successful strategy flow from our analysis of
the dynamics of health agencies. The first and cardinal ground-rule is
that a change strategy must recognise the local dimension in the NHS.
A prescription that applies equally to all health agencies will not do.
The things that will make for development or hinder it in Exeter are
not present in exactly the same form in Newcastle. The instruments of
change, therefore, must discriminate between different areas of the
country.

The second ground-rule is that the strategy must recognise the likely
predominance of the local political system in decision-making. Arrangements predicated on the normality of the rational decision-making
models will not, therefore, have much impact. This is why the NHS
planning system does not meet this second ground-rule. It meets the
first, because the focus of attention is the local strategic and operational plans and they will reflect different local conditions. However,
the strength of the local impulses to act politically to advance particular values and interests will diminish the impact of rational analysis
(if such a state of grace were possible to achieve, which it is not). The
planning system will thus provide the arenas and language for the
political process rather than change its nature. A change strategy must
therefore influence the local political systems directly to effect readier
responses to changes in circumstances.

The third ground-rule is the recognition of the true function of management in the NHS. Strategies based on the notion that top managers
have a directing role, and impulses for change can thus be routed
through them, are bound to fail. Managers in the NHS are not the most
powerful group, and therefore have not the control assumed in classical
organisational theory (and probably never can, given the 'democratisation' of society). In the case of the NHS, providers are more central to
its functioning and managers are more dependent on them rather than
vice versa. Change strategies must, therefore, be directed at the total
local system for management and *not* managers: they remain only one
part of that system, and possibly one of the least powerful.

This is not to say that all ideas associated with scientific management should be discarded, for such a course would be foolish. It is a

plea for recognition of the fact that the power of managers in the NHS
to effect change is very limited and that the ideology they represent
does not fit easily with that of providers. The priority managers and
providers would accord to the right design of organisation (i.e. tidy
hierarchial arrangements, with responsibilities neatly defined and par-
celled out) will differ. It is not that either group necessarily disagrees
with it in principle. Rather, they ascribe a different priority to this
feature of organisational life, as the retreat from the hierarchal notions
in the arrangements for the organisation of medical work since 1974
has demonstrated. The continuing tensions associated with the Salmon
management structure for nurses is another example of differences of
view about appropriate structure at work. The priority accorded to this
aspect of the nursing function is higher among the profession's leaders
than it is among the practitioners.

Similarly, other features of the management philosophy such as
methods of decision-making and the priority attached to the criteria of
economy and efficiency may not generate the same enthusiasm among
all groups of providers, even if there was general assent to the basic
propositions. It might be argued that the change strategy should be
directed to encouraging providers to accord these particular features of
managerialism a higher priority in their own behaviour. There is much
to be said for that point of view. However, the thrust of the argument
here is that the change is not best effected by using managers as the
instruments of change: they have not the 'clout' to do it.

A fourth requirement is orientation to the end product of the services and not the levels of input, or the subtleties of different organisational arrangements. The planning system was designed to effect this
change of emphasis but the norms of provision, guidelines and priorities
remain obstinately concerned with the level of provision rather than
what it achieves in terms of the welfare of the patient. In contrast, the
productive debate on the best type of maternity care in the context of
infant mortality and handicap is an illustration of what can be achieved.
The strategy for change should aim to generalise preoccupation with
ends rather than means.

There may be other ingredients, equally or perhaps more essential to
an effective strategy for change in the NHS than described here. These
are the ones that flow from our argument and material on health
agencies, but we have made it clear that much more needs to be known
about the dynamics of the NHS. Our analysis is one of the first steps
into these particular waters and the list of essential ingredients cannot
be offered as an exhaustive one. It nevertheless offers a starting point

from which to fashion better ways of helping health agencies make necessary changes in a ready and responsive manner. The strategy must be agency specific; act directly on elements and actors in the local political system to encourage these most responsive to changes in circumstances; it must not depend on the power of managers for its initiation and support; and it should direct attention to the impact of services on health and welfare of patients.

This last element in a successful change strategy makes an appropriate final point for the book, since it directs our attention to patients. The situation in which local managers and providers have found themselves has not encouraged them to think of outputs and health outcomes: the emphasis has been on the inputs and their inadequacy. The central department, to its credit, has been more aware of the longer-term economic, social and medical changes that would change the balance of local tasks. It has, no doubt, been stimulated by the growing concern with the effectiveness and direction of public services, including the NHS. The failure of the centre to find adequate ways and means of effecting adequate responses to this growing concern from its agents in the field does not mean that the task should be abandoned. The threat to the NHS posed by current economic conditions and the growth of private medicine strengthens the case for almost total preoccupation with what the service *actually* does for the welfare of the patients. Otherwise, the 'collapse' of the NHS, forecasted by many for years past, might become a reality.

Notes

1. See, for example, Lord Taylor of Harlow, 'Health Services for the Eighties', *World Medicine*, vol. 14, no. 17 (1979).

2. See, for example, H. Clegg, *Trade Unionism under Collective Bargaining* (Blackwell, Oxford, 1976).

3. D. Hunter, 'Coping with Uncertainty: Decisions and Resources within Health Authorities', *Sociology of Health and Illness*, vol. 1, no. 1 (1979).

4. M. Rein, *Social Science and Public Policy* (Penguin, Harmondsworth, 1976).

5. Royal Commission on the National Health Service, *Report*, Cmnd. 7615 (HMSO, London, 1979). See particularly paras. 12.38 to 12.43.

6. Ibid., paras. 15.23 to 15.32.

7. B. Smith, *Policy Making in British Government* (Martin Robertson, London, 1976), p. 16.

8. S. Lukes, *Power – A Radical View* (Macmillan, London, 1974), p. 15.

9. Ibid., p. 19. This extract is based on the work of P. Bachrach and M.S. Barat, *Power and Poverty, Theory and Practice* (Oxford University Press, New York, 1970).

10. Ibid., p. 23.

11. Ibid., p. 24.

12. G. Best, J. Dennis and P. Draper, *Health, the Mass Media and the National Health Service* (Unit for the Study of Health Policy, 1976), p. 28.

13. Ibid., p. 33.

14. V. Navarro, *Class Struggle, the State and Medicine* (Martin Robertson, London, 1978), and *Medicine under Capitalism* (Croom Helm, London, 1976).

15. See especially National Union of Public Employees, *Good Health* (NUPE, 1978).

16. Central Health Services Council, *The Functions of the District General Hospital*, Report of the Committee (HMSO, London 1969).

17. DHSS, *Better Services for the Mentally Handicapped*, Cmnd. 4683 (HMSO, London, 1971).

18. Committee of Enquiry into Mental Handicap Nursing and Care, *Report*, Chairman, P. Jay, vol. 1, Cmnd. 7468-1 (HMSO, London, 1979).

19. S. Dimmock and K. Barnard, 'Relationships and Communications' in E. Raybould (ed.), *A Guide for Nurse Managers* (Blackwell, Oxford, 1977), p. 102.

20. Hunter, 'Coping with Uncertainty'.

21. H.J. Elcock and S.C. Haywood with T.L. Jones, *Research Report* on Decentralised Administration in the NHS. For the Social Science Research Council, University of Hull, 1980.

22. A Strauss *et al.*, 'The Hospital and its Negotiated Order' in F.G. Castles *et al., Decisions, Organisations and Society* (Penguin Education, Harmondsworth, 1971), pp. 103-4.

23. Hunter, 'Coping with Uncertainty'.

24. R. Greenwood, C.R. Hinings and S. Ranson, *The Politics of the Budgetary Process in English Local Government*, paper presented to a Political Studies Association Conference, Nottingham, March 1976.

25. For a concise summary see, *The Administrative Process as Incrementalism* (The Open University Press, 1974).

26. Ibid., p. 73.

27. DHSS and Welsh Office, *Patients First* (HMSO, London, 1979).

28. E. Powell, *Medicine and Politics* (Pitman Medical, 1966), pp. 15-16.

29. Royal Commission on the National Health Service, *Report*, Cmnd. 7615 (HMSO, London, 1979), para. 21.4.

30. Ibid., para. 22. 81.

31. See, for example, A.L. Cochrane, *Effectiveness and Efficiency* (Nuffield Provincial Hospital Trust, London, 1971).

32. For a discussion of this problem, see K.M. Boyd, *The Ethics of Resource Allocation in Health Care* (Edinburgh University Press, 1979).

33. S.C. Haywood *et al., The Curate's Egg . . . Good in Parts. Senior Officer Reflections on the NHS* (Institute for Health Studies, University of Hull, 1979).

34. D. Schon, *Beyond the Stable State* (Penguin, Harmondsworth, 1973).

35. *Sunday Telegraph*, news story, 21 October 1979.

INDEX